BrainPower

Tools and Tips for Mental Sharpness,

Improved Memory, and

A Better Life—No Matter How Old You Are

By Dr. Chris E. Stout, PsyD.

Clinical Professor, College of Medicine, University of Illinois

Associate Professor, Northwestern University Feinberg School of Medicine

Post-Doctoral Fellow, Harvard Medical School

Table of Contents

Endorsements

Dedication

Foreword

Chapter 1: Introduction

Chapter 2: The Utility of Having a Diagnosis

Chapter 3: Memory: Getting Sharp and Staying Sharp

Chapter 4: Breaking Bad Habits

Chapter 5: Supplements and Nutraceuticals

Chapter 6: Medications and Pharmaceuticals

Chapter 7: Diet: You are What You Eat

Chapter 8: Physical Exercise

Chapter 9: Purpose and Quality of Life

Appendix and Additional Resources

Appendix A: Functional Activities Questionnaire (FAQ)

Appendix B: Extended Personal Inventory

Glossary

References and Resources

Books

Articles

Websites and Organizations

Author's Biography

Endorsements

"As we live longer, our biggest concern will be the health of our minds. We can always use a wheelchair, but life's not much use if you don't know where to wheel yourself. *BrainPower* provides provocative insights and action steps to keep us firing on all cylinders." *Dr. Mehmet Oz, MD, MBA, FACS*

> *Dr. Mehmet Oz is one of the most respected surgeons in the world, as well as host of Second Opinion on the Discovery Health Channel. He is the Irving Associate Professor of Cardiac Surgery at Columbia University, directs the Hear Assist Device Program and is a founder of the Complementary Medicine Program at New York Presbyterian Medical Center. He has authored more than 350 original publications, book chapters, abstracts, and books and has received several patents. Dr. Oz received his undergraduate degree from Harvard University (1982) and obtained a joint MD and MBA (1986) from the University of Pennsylvania School of Medicine and Wharton Business School.*

"*BrainPower* is a truly remarkable, must needed effort, the authors have assembled a formidable weapon against cognitive/memory affecting scourges like Alzheimer's Disease or other dementias, as well as disorders resulting in severe learning difficulties in our children."
Dr. Ronald F. Levant, EdD, ABPP, MBA

> *Dr. Ronald F. Levant, current president of the American Psychological Association, received his doctrate in Clinical Psychology and Public Practice from Harvard University. More recently, he obtained an MBA with high honors from Boston University. Dr. Levant, Dean and Professor of Psychology at the Buchel College of Arts and Sciences, University of Akron, has served on the faculty of Boston, Rutgers, and Harvard Universities. He has authored and edited more than 250 publications, including 14 books, more than 140 peer-reviewed journal articles, book chapters in family and male psychology, and more than 70 newsletter columns. He has served as the editor of the Journal of Family Psychology (1992-1997), guest editor for special issues of the following journals: The Counseling Psychologist, Journal of Clinical Psychology in Medical Settings, and the Journal of African American Men, has been on the editorial boards of 11 journals and is currently the associate editor for Professional Psychology: Research and Practice. Dr. Levant has been interviewed for hundreds of articles in such publications as Fortune, Industry Week, Newsweek, Time, U.S. News and World Report, People Magazine, The Boston Globe, The New York Times, Christian Science Monitor, USA Today, Wall Street Journal, Associated Press, and United Press International. He has appeared on numerous national television shows including "20/20", "The Oprah Winfrey Show", and "CBS News Nightline".*

BrainPower is..."An engaging, scientifically based, yet highly practical approach describing what we can do for ourselves and our loved ones, as our Nation's population steadily matures. Oftentimes confusing medical jargon is straightforwardly explained with useful and understandable advice proffered. Suggestions for daily exercises and dietary modifications are especially helpful."
Dr. Patrick DeLeon, PhD, JD, MBA

> *Dr. DeLeon, recent Past President of the American Psychological Association, is the first recipient of the Hawaii Psychological Association's Lifetime Achievement Award. Dr. DeLeon has been on the staff of Senator Daniel K. Inoye (D-Hawaii) since 1974. His career has been marked by significant legislative achievement, including establishing the emergency medical service system, which helps emergency rooms provide the best possible physical and psychosocial care for children.*

"*BrainPower* pulls together all the very latest advances in the science of keeping well, integrating knowledge from a huge range of disciplines and resources, the authors provide the best possible basis for improving our sense of well-being at whatever age. In particular, its innovative approach to memory and the mind makes it highly relevant for aging baby boomers looking to keep their cognitive edge."

Dr. Margaret Hannah, MB, M-chir, FFPHM

Dr. Margaret Hannah graduated in medicine from Cambridge University and St. Thomas's Hospital Medical School in 1986. She practiced general medicine in London and Hong Kong, until making the transition into public health in 1991. She completed public health training in London and was appointed a Consultant in Public Health Medicine in 1996. Her areas of expertise include mental health, addiction services, and providing advice on the development of local health improvement programs. Dr. Hannah has been involved in the Healthy Public Policy Network (an independent think tank) since 1997 and has contributed to numerous publications in the process, currently working on a national project examining the mental health needs of children and young people.

Dedication

To my family, Karen, Grayson, and Annika, for being so ever-tolerant of my missing-in-action during the production of this book.

Foreword

The International Longevity Center states that even without new scientific breakthroughs people in industrialized countries could increase their lifespan "at least 10-years" by eating less and exercising more: "Half the [U.S.] population is overweight, 20% are obese, and only 15% of people over the age of 65 regularly exercise. Our diets are overwhelmingly conducive to the development of heart disease, and far too many of us still use tobacco products." Staying mentally, physically and emotionally fit is the key to having "BrainPower."

It is not that research does not exist, or even that techniques, medications, and clinical approaches are missing for Alzheimer's disease and other dementias or memory problems. What has been missing, however, is a resource where peer-reviewed studies from various professions are summarized in a readable, accessible, understandable, and actionable single source—that is until this book.

Evidence-based practice and practice-based evidence have been brought together in these volumes in such a way as to provide readers with a strong basis for understanding the complex and often confounding world of intellectual decline, confusion, loss of focus, concentration and memory impairments, debilitating problems that are often attached to dreaded diagnoses like Alzheimer's Disease, Autistic Spectrum Disorders, Attention Deficit Disorders (ADD/ADHD), Dyslexia, and a myriad of other Learning Disabilities too numerous to name.

Eric M. Reiman, writing on Alzheimer's Disease in *The Journal of Clinical Psychiatry*, notes that "even a modestly effective prevention therapy could have an enormous impact [and that] delaying the onset of Alzheimer's Disease by only 5 years could reduce the number of afflicted patients by half" (66:7, 2005, p. 816).

Regrettably, no one can guarantee that all readers and users of the recommendations contained in these books will never suffer from Alzheimer's or other cognitive disabilities, ADHD or other types of learning disabilities, and/or Pervasive Developmental Disorders. Having said that, for those who do what is recommended herein, based on the author's research of the literature (evidence-based practice) and clinical work (practice-based evidence), the quality of their lives will definitely be enhanced, and significantly so for many.

Chapter 1

Introduction

Current Status and Concerns

Each generation in the United States lives longer, accounting for an average three year increase in life expectancy since the beginning of the twentieth century. Unfortunately, the price we pay for living longer is an increased risk of developing typically "late-life" disorders such as cancer, arthritis, heart disease and dementia. Among the most feared of these conditions (almost equal to the fear of cancer) is that of Alzheimer's Disease (AD) which, like all dementing illnesses, severely affects memory, attention, and concentration. Concerns about such illnesses impact not only those at risk, but their loved ones as well. It is currently estimated that within the near future, the incidence of AD could increase by a staggering 70% to approximately 14 million individuals.

The good news is that there is a growing body of scientific, evidence-based literature highlighting treatments intended to prevent, delay, and/or diminish the effects of Alzheimer's Disease dementing illnesses. This book is a compilation of such evidence-based data, combined with an integrated model for diagnosis and treatment. The model includes a proprietary, state of the art assessment which leads to individualized remedial treatment. "Individualized" means that the model targets deficits within specific areas of a given individual's brain and develops personalized learning programs to improve functioning in those areas.

The Model and Method

The purpose of **BrainPower**$^{(TM)}$ is to provide clear, concise, reader-friendly yet research-based information needed in order to avoid, postpone, and/or minimize symptoms of memory loss and intellectual decline while promoting physical and emotional well-being. The chapters in these books offer guidelines as to what you or your loved one can start doing today to help with improving memory, thinking, cognitive abilities, and emotional abilities. In other words, you now have a complete, detailed review of the clinical, scientific, and medical literature. This book has compiled a vast literature into the chapters of these books—all volumes for way less than the cost of one fill-up of gas. Really!

Although the focus of these books deal with dementing illnesses, these volumes are equally concerned with Attention Deficit Disorders (ADHD), Dyslexia, Autistic Spectrum Disorders (including Asperser's Syndrome), and other Learning or Pervasive Developmental Disorders, minimizing the effects of aging, enhancing athletic abilities, and emotional stability.

Differential Diagnoses of Dementia

Although Alzheimer's Disease (AD) is a leading cause of dementia, other causes and coexisting conditions are being recognized more frequently. The table below lists changes associated with several types of dementia:

Dementia Type	Typical Presentation
Mild Cognitive Impairment (MCI)	A relatively new term which suggests that a person shows some but not all of the signs of dementia and these symptoms are not yet too so severe (this category is also known more commonly as Age Related Cognitive Decline)
Alzheimer's Disease (AD)	Impaired recent memory, word finding, general intellect, visuospatial processing, memory recognition, and apraxia, all developing insidiously over years
Vascular Dementia (formerly called multi-infarct Dementia)	General intellectual decline over time, memory disturbance, executive dysfunction, apathy and/or motivation: possible gait disturbance, visual field loss, and focal findings becoming manifest and worsening in a step-wise fashion
Dementia with Lewy Bodies or Lewy Body Disease	Fluctuating cognition with pronounced variation in attention and alertness, recurrent detailed visual hallucinations, spontaneous motor features of parkinsonism, sensitivity to neuroleptic medication
Parkinson's Dementia	Memory preserved early, later impaired speech marked by hypophonia and dysarthria, hesitation, apathy, irritable and depressive features
Frontotemporal Dementia	Changes in personality, executive function, and behavior, apathy, disinhibition, labile affect, irritability, and assaultiveness; relatively preserved memory until later in course of illness
Normal Pressure Hydrocephalus (NPH)	Feeling that one's feet are glued to the floor (leading to shuffling when walking), urinary incontinence, mild memory loss

* Greenstein, S., Davidson, H. E. Eds. A Pocket Guide to Dementia and Associated Behavioral Symptoms: Diagnosis, Assessment and Management. Second Edition, 2003. Reprinted with permission of Insight Therapies, LLC.

Several additional forms of Dementia not listed in the chart above include: Mixed Dementia (e.g. a combination of AD and vascular dementia), Dementia Syndrome of Depression (or *Pseudodementia*), Prion Diseases, Traumatic Brain Injuries, Non-degenerative, Nonvascular Dementias, and Cognitive Disorder NOS (Not Otherwise

Specified), a catchall category for when there is insufficient information to clearly indicate the type of dementing illness.

To fully benefit from the recommendations contained in this book, some of you may have several long-standing bad habits to break first and that may be a challenge. Others of you will only need to make minor adjustments to certain aspects of your lifestyle. Still others will need to craft a comprehensive new way of life for the future. No matter where you are, this book will help by serving as a tool to guide you as you make these changes. Let us get started with additional background information and try to answer some questions you may have.

Frequently Asked Questions (And With Answers!) About Memory Loss

1) *How prevalent is Alzheimer's Disease or AD?*

It is currently estimated that at least four million Americans suffer from Alzheimer's Disease, making it the most common form of dementing illness, accounting for more than 65% of all dementing illnesses in the elderly. By the year 2050, it is estimated that the number will increase to at least 14 million and may be even closer to that number now than previously believed.

2) *Why is Alzheimer's Disease seen as such a problem?*

At an annual cost for the four million current sufferers of $90 billion for medical care, social services, and lost productivity, Alzheimer's remains one of the most expensive diseases to manage, notwithstanding the devastating emotional toll for the person as well as his or her loved ones and caregivers.

3) *Are men or women more likely to get Alzheimer's Disease?*

Alzheimer's Disease is twice as common in men as women.

4) *Are there other memory illnesses?*

Yes, as indicated by our earlier table, there are a number of other causes of memory loss. The second most common disease of memory loss and intellectual impairment, for example, is called "Lewy Body Dementia" (or LBD). "Lewy bodies" are regions of your brain that may deteriorate as a result of aging or the onset of Parkinson's disease.

5) *My doctor has mentioned "Vascular dementias." What are those?*

Vascular types of dementia are the third most frequent cause of memory problems and are most common in men over 70 years of age. However, they can also occur much earlier in individuals with a history of high blood pressure, diabetes, and/or significant alcohol, street drug or tobacco use. This type of memory loss is most commonly associated with strokes (often referred to medically as cerebrovascular accidents [CVAs] and/or transient ischemic attacks [TIAs]). Both often, but not always, result in damage to the brain that can be observed on Computerized Tomography (CT) scans and/or Magnetic Resonance Imagery (MRI).

6)   *Can diseases affecting memory be inherited?*

Diseases such as Pick's Disease, Cruetzfeldt-Jakob Disease, and Wilson's Disease (also known collectively as "Prion Diseases") have a strong genetic predisposition of which most individuals and their physicians should be aware. Consequently, such diseases can usually be diagnosed earlier than other dementing illnesses.

7)   *If I get hit in the head, will I get amnesia?*

It's certainly possible, though not as likely as TV sitcoms would have you believe. Memory loss can occur as a result of traumatic injuries to the brain such as concussions, open head wounds, and even persistent and significant alcohol and/or drug abuse.

8)   *What about excessive alcohol consumption or the use/abuse of other drugs like cocaine, marijuana, ecstasy, LSD, etc.?*

Alcohol and other drugs can severely traumatize the brain, which often leads to emotional and cognitive impairment as well as general medical decline.

9)   *I have been diagnosed with Major Depression, but it seems like I also have a problem with my memory.*

It sounds like you might have Dementia Syndrome of Depression, or *Pseudodementia*, as it was originally known. Memory loss secondary to clinical depression is more correctly diagnosed simply as depression, since clinically depressed individuals often show reduced cognitive abilities (attention, memory, concentration, focus, recall) due to their depressed mood state as opposed to a dementing illness. However, certain key diagnostic considerations and assessments help to rule out the presence of a co-occurring, true dementia.

10)   *How is Pseudodementia treated?*

The most effective treatment for *Pseudodementia* or Dementia Syndrome of Depression involves a combination of anti-depressant medication and Cognitive-Behavioral Therapy.

11)   *My child has been diagnosed with a Learning Disability and with a short-term memory deficit. Is there anything to help him?*

Memory is composed of three sections – short-term, working, and long-term. Several techniques can be utilized to improve memory functioning, including several in this book.

12)   *The medical community states the number of children with Autism and Autism Spectrum Disorders is growing. Can a child with Autism improve their interactions?*

Individuals with these disorders have poor nonverbal behavior that may be remediated through specific programs with reinforcement systems.

13)   *Does childhood Attention Deficit Hyperactivity Disorder (ADD/ADHD) continue into adulthood?*

The answer is yes, with impairments manifested in academic, professional/employment, emotionally, and socially. Adult ADHD is also under diagnosed and under treated.

"Senior Moments" Are No Laughing Matter

The cliché about having a forgetful or "senior moment" has become such a common part of our collective experience that it is quickly, almost jokingly recognized as an inability to remember something like a person's name, a phone number, or even where you just left your car keys or reading glasses. At first, if done in the company of others, such incidents can be a source of good-natured ribbing. Over time, however, such memory "glitches" become less humorous as they worsen and/or become more frequent.

The good news is that sufficient scientific data is now available to allow for an integrated, holistic, and research-based system that can help avoid or at least postpone intellectual decline in your mental/cognitive/memory/executive abilities. For some, seeking professional healthcare consultation and treatment may be necessary if problems have progressed too far along. This book is NOT meant to serve as a substitute for professional healthcare services; instead, it is an adjunctive tool to help you maintain, if not *improve*, your current level of cognitive ability – memory, focus, concentration, emotional-coping and stress management skills for a richer, more satisfying, and "independent" life.

Chapter 2

The Utility of Having a Diagnosis

A diagnosis is a description of a condition a person has. It is made up of a group of symptoms, which have been associated with a specific type of disease, illness, or condition. The utility of a diagnosis lies in summarizing the results of examinations, such as those discussed earlier, and then communicating the findings in "shorthand" to other professionals.

In the mental health field, diagnostic criteria (symptoms) are collected and arranged in a book called the Diagnostic and Statistical Manual of Mental Disorders, Fourth Edition (DSM-IV-R™). The diagnostic process is constantly being revised and updated by standing committees in the mental health professions to reflect the progress of research and practice over time.

Diagnostic Process of Cognitive Impairment

Many people wonder what is involved in determining a diagnosis of, for example, dementia or Alzheimer's. Historically, the following have been the most likely components in formatting a diagnosis:

- complete Medical History (including histories of psychiatric and/or substance abuse histories and past head trauma)

- Neuropsychological Testing

- complete blood cell count

- serum electrolytes

- blood glucose, blood urea, and certainties

- serum Vitamin B-12 levels

- depression screening

- liver function tests

- brain scan (such as CT or MRI)

It is also advisable that you visit your healthcare professional with a loved one or trusted friend who can take notes, ask questions you may not have considered, and to fill in any gaps in your history, which you may accidentally omit. Some tests (like the Mini-Mental State Exam, RBans, etc) may do double duty by establishing a baseline for ongoing comparison.

Screening Approaches

As will be discussed later in this chapter, there are also a number of other screening techniques that may be helpful to know about, and/or try. Of course, these are NOT substitutes for a comprehensive work-up by a healthcare specialist.

The Critical Use of Diagnosis in Aging

As you will see in an upcoming section on "Differentiating the 3 D's of Cognitive Impairment," in diagnosing dementia one must distinguish it from delirium and depression (e.g. also called *Pseudodementia*). Further, it is important to distinguish between different types of dementia because treatment options and outcomes are specific to each category.

Try This (CAREFULLY) At Home

Close your eyes, lift one foot off the ground, and count how long you can hold that position. It may seem simple, but balance is a great measure of cerebellar functioning. The longer the time, the better. Here is the general scale for men:

Age (in years)	Expected Time (in seconds)
20 – 30	~28
31 – 40	~23
41 – 60	~15

"Sniff" Test

Difficulties smelling have also been associated with Alzheimer's disease. The biological systems involved are the parts of the brain associated with the perception of odors. These regions are destroyed due to beta-amyloid plaques that build up in the brains of Alzheimer's patients and block the flow of blood and oxygen. According to some researchers, there is a greater likelihood for people to develop Alzheimer's if they cannot detect the following odors:

Strawberry	Smoke
Soap	Menthol
Clove	Pineapple
Natural Gas	Lilac

Lemon	Leather

There are even "smell tests" currently available based on this new research.

Medications That May Negatively Impact Memory

In determining an accurate diagnosis, it is important to judge whether other factors may be the actual cause of the problem. For example, there are a number of medications that can in and of themselves interfere with cognitive functioning. Similarly, some medications can deplete vitamin and mineral levels which then negatively impact memory functioning. A detailed listing of these medications is contained in Chapter Six.

Medical Conditions That May Negatively Impact Memory

A number of medical illnesses or conditions can also adversely affect memory and cognitive functions. The following table notes many of the more common ones:

Medical Problem	Examples
Hormonal Imbalances	Thyroid disease
	Cushing's disease
Infectious Diseases	AIDS
	Syphilis
	Chronic meningitis
Tumors	Frontal lobe
	Temporal lobe
Trauma	Subdural hematoma
Vitamin deficiencies	Limited intake of Vitamin B-12
Heavy metal toxicity	Lead or mercury poisoning
Normal-pressure hydrocephalus	Excess fluid in the brain

The Importance of Differentiating Between the Three Ds of Cognitive Impairment: Delirium, Dementia, and Depression

These three disorders may manifest with very similar symptoms of memory and cognitive impairment. It is critical that an experienced health professional (such as a neuropsychologist) first clinically differentiate which is the primary cause of cognitive malfunction before proceeding, ensuring the appropriate treatment plan is chosen. The following table may be used in the meantime to help you better understand the differences (adapted with permission from Rabins, P. V. The Memory Bulletin, Spring 2005, Johns Hopkins School of Medicine: Baltimore, MD, p. 24, 1/28/05).

Feature	Delirium	Dementia	Depression
Onset	Sudden (hours to days), with an identifiable time of onset	Gradual (months to year) with no identifiable time of onset	Rapid (weeks to months)
Duration/Progression	Usually hours to days: reversible with successful treatment	Remainder of patient's life; typically worsens over time despite treatment	Usually short term, but persistent in some people; reversible with successful treatment
Psychiatric History	Often no previous psychiatric problems	Often no previous psychiatric problems	Usually has a history of psychiatric problems, including undiagnosed episodes of depression
General deficits	Displays new deficits	May try to hide any new deficits	Acknowledges new deficits
Memory	Rapid fluctuations; difficulty recalling recent events	Memory for recent events and common knowledge slowly erodes but is relatively stable day to day; often unaware of memory loss	Occasional fluctuations in performance; recognizes and is troubled by forgetfulness
Thinking	Disorganized; may be sluggish or racing	Difficulty with abstract ideas word finding calculations, judgment, recognition	Fluctuating problems
Alertness/attention	Inattentiveness and drowsiness a concern	Usually normal; may attend to one idea for a prolonged period	Generally reduced; difficulty concentrating
Language	Often incoherent, rapid or slow, and slurred	Often incoherent; difficulty finding correct words	Slow; difficulty attending to a conversation

Answers to questions	Often incoherent and rambling	Responds incorrectly with near misses	Often responds with "I don't know"
Mood	Unstable, with rapid swings	Fluctuates; may show apathy, depression	Extreme sadness, often with anxiety or irritability
Activity level	Hyperactive or sluggish (may fluctuate between the to); tremors or spasms	Normal at first, but decreases late in the disease	Lethargic, restless, or agitated
Sleep/wake cycle	Disturbed with variations from hour to hour; sleep/wake cycles may be reversed	Disturbed, often with a reversal of day/night sleep cycle	Insomnia (difficulty falling asleep or early-morning waking) or excessive sleep
Awareness of Deficit	Often unaware	Often unaware	Often exaggerates the perceived deficits

A health care professional usually screens for dementia when there are reported cognitive changes such as memory loss or disorientation; psychiatric symptoms or other mental health signs that have to do with cognition, perception, mood, changes in personality (paranoia, explosive anger without a prior history of these behaviors) and changes in daily functioning including declines in IADLs - Instrumental Activities of Daily Living (see Appendix A for a sample Functional Activities Questionnaire).

Individuals and their loved ones should consider a comprehensive evaluation if one or more of the following changes occur (adapted from Rabins et al (1999):

Cognitive changes – recent forgetfulness, increased difficulty understanding spoken and written communication, difficulty finding words, not knowing things the person should know, disorientation, spouse or caregiver is forced to answer all questions in clinical interviews.

Psychiatric symptoms – social withdrawal, depression, anxiety, insomnia, paranoia, abnormal beliefs, hallucinations, delusions, irritability.

Personality changes – inappropriate friendliness, apathy, rapid emotional mood shifts, social withdrawal, excessive flirtatiousness, low tolerance leading to frustration, suspiciousness, disinhibition, development of uncharacteristic or inappropriate traits, intensification of premorbid traits.

Problem behaviors – wandering, noisiness, restlessness, being out of bed at night, catastrophic reactions, explosive spells, recklessness, carelessness; verbal or physical agitation or aggression.

Changes in day-to-day functioning (IADLs – instrumental activities of daily living) – difficulty driving, handling money, shopping neglecting self-care, hygiene (grooming, eating, etc.), household chores, getting lost, making mistakes at work or with bills, missing appointments. Further examples of IADLs include:

1. Writing checks, paying bills, balancing a checkbook

2. Assembling tax records, business affairs, or papers

3. Shopping alone for clothes, house-hold necessities, or groceries

4. Playing a game of skill, working on a hobby

5. Heating water, making a cup of coffee, turning off the stove

6. Preparing a balanced meal, keeping track of current events

7. Paying attention to, under-standing, discussing a TV show, book, or magazine

8. Remembering appointments, family occasions, holidays, medications

9. Traveling out of the neighborhood, driving, arranging to take buses

Here is a diagnostic pop quiz. Joe is becoming confused; his wife has noticed memory loss, bizarre thinking, depressed mood, irritability and aggression, and loss of mobility and balance. She's also noticed sudden changes in Joe's ability to control his bowel and bladder. She thinks Joe has dementia. Is she right? Should she be looking for a safe environment for him to live in? Not necessarily. In this case, Joe may actually have a medical condition that is easily treated, even though his symptoms at first glance may suggest dementia.

You see, Joe is also exhibiting all the symptoms of Low Pressure Hydrocephalus or water build up in and around the brain that causes cognitive changes or memory loss and confusion, bizarre thinking, depression, irritability, aggression, loss of balance and changes in gait (walking), and incontinence of bowel and/or bladder. The usual treatment includes the surgical insertion of an intracranial "shunt" (a tube placed into the skull) to relieve the pressure that has built up so that the individual returns to their usual self in a matter of days. Joe's problem and effective treatment plan are reasons why we must remind you once again that a quick "test" or "quiz" on the internet or in your favorite magazine is no substitute for a complete evaluation by an appropriately trained/experienced professional.

Intercranial bleeding, usually caused by a subdural hematoma (bleeding under the duramatter of the skull) also has similar adverse effects on all aspects of functioning. If the treating professional orders a scan (CT, MRI) of the brain, they should be able to see the changes resulting from pressure that has built up to a point that is detrimental to the individual's functioning. Sadly, these tests are not always ordered for the elderly as a diagnosis of dementia can also be made and much less expensively, even if not always as accurately, based on the presenting symptoms alone.

Nowhere is this more clearly illustrated than in the area of brain problems, including memory difficulties in general, as well as any of the dementias. Yearly neuropsychological testing for age-related cognitive performance starting around age 60 or earlier (depending on the number and severity of symptoms both physical and cognitive) would greatly increase the likelihood of successful diagnosis in the event of a sudden change in cognitive status.

Neuroplasticity

In the last decade, great strides have been made in brain research and treatment. For example, researchers originally thought that the brain's nerve cells, called neurons, were both specialized and unable to regenerate. We now know that brain cells can be grown from common precursors and that they can regenerate. That's more good news for those who are aging and who have concerns about memory loss or other problems.

The concept of neuroplasticity states that the brain can rewire, renew, and regenerate itself in response to trauma or stress (e.g. damage, disease and/or dysfunction), in ways that were not understood or even anticipated a number of years ago. Neuroplasticity underscores the brains ability to adapt to insult or injury and to find alternative routes with which to realize its functional capacity, in spite of the damage.

Children and Neuroplasticity

Neuroplasticity is even more important for children since their brains have been shown to be more malleable or "plastic" than the fully developed adult brain. Thus, a child who sustains a brain injury is more likely to make a significant or full recovery because his brain is still developing. By the way, although the brain stops growing externally in size by around age 16, it continues to "grow" internally by forming dense neural pathways throughout the lifespan. Exactly how does such growth occur? Growth occurs through activity, exercise, and proper nutrition. The old saying is true: "if you don't use it, you lose it," even for children.

Any discussion about children and brain development should include how primary cognitive skills develop. The skills necessary for social life, as some researchers like Russell Barkley suggest, are listed in the chart below:

Nonverbal Working Memory	Verbal Working Memory	Emotional Regulation	Planning and Organization
Develops at birth	Develops with the onset of speech	Present at birth, more skill with speech onset	Develops with concept of time management
Attention	Holding items in memory	Moods are managed to fit the needs of the situation	Awareness of time needed to finish a task
Concentration	Recalling items in memory	Responsiveness to emotional feedback	View of scheduling 8-12 weeks ahead as an adult
Visual Focus	Remembering to complete an action	Responsiveness to consequences	View of scheduling 8-12 weeks ahead as an adult
Visual Recognition	Remembering a series of items	Empathy and empathic responses	
Imitation	Preparing information for long-term storage	Empathy and empathic responses	Views the schedule 8-12 weeks ahead as an adult
Vicarious Learning or learning from others' mistakes	Development of useable encoding strategies for multi-step directions	Moods are managed to fit the needs of the situation	Plans and organizes behaviors to meet goals in the distant future

* Adapted and modified from a presentation on Attention Deficit Hyperactivity Disorders: Etiology and Theory by Russell A. Barkley, PhD. 2005

If these brain based skills do not develop fully, the child may eventually be diagnosed with Autism, Asperser's Syndrome or some other Pervasive Developmental Disorder, Mental Retardation, a Learning Disability (Reading, Math, Written Language, Nonverbal Learning Disorder), or Attention Deficit Disorder (with or without Hyperactivity). It is important to note that in the real world, a child may not be organized, plan particularly well, or be sufficiently sensitive or empathic and yet function at a high level both personally and socially. However, if that same child has poorly developed nonverbal skills, they will not function as well. Furthermore, they will be more likely to be identified as having developmental or other disorders. For example the difference between the diagnosis for Autism and ADHD is that individuals with Autism are usually identified much earlier because the child does not develop "age appropriate" nonverbal skills.

Diagnostic Procedures

Here is a list of some available diagnostic procedures and treatments for ADD/ADHD.

1. *Brain scans.* MRI studies by Dan Amen and his group have shown some promise, but the research is not conclusive as of yet.
2. *Behavior Charts.* Rating scales of the level and frequency of the child's

misbehaviors. Such scales are usually subjective rather than objective, which can increase error rates, where raters also commonly disagree about the frequency, duration, and intensity of the behavior being rated based on their specific relationship with the child.

3. *Psychological/Neuropsychological Testing.* Regrettably, insurance companies seldom pay for what they refer to as "Psychoeducational Testing," which unfortunately includes tests for assessing the symptoms of ADD/ADHD and other learning disabilities. That is because if it is primarily educationally related, they argue that the school psychologist (a related but separate specialty from clinical psychology) should be doing the testing (at the taxpayer's expense rather than the insurance company's). Appropriately trained clinicians use specific measures designed to gather relevant histories, and measure common comorbid (co-occurring) disorders. Unfortunately, children (and adults) with ADD/ADHD are significantly more likely to be diagnosed with multiple problems such as other learning disabilities (50% of all cases). Depression and/or anxiety (25% of all cases) and other conditions such as oppositional/defiant behavior disorder, conduct disorder, and bipolar disorder.

4. *Head Movement.* Systems of measuring an individual's head movements as continuous performance tasks are completed. Measures hyperkinetic behavior.

More Treatment Options

1. *Stimulant Medication.* Still the primary treatment for ADD/ADHD, and despite all the concerns about these medications, there is existing research that the medical community is underprescribing them based on international prevalence studies.

2. *Dietary Changes.* Works by eliminating artificial sweeteners, eating only organically grown foods, eliminating yellow dyes, and diet programs such as the Feingold Diet, Nature's Cure, etc.

3. *Nutraceutical Therapy.* A healthy diet, pharmaceutical grade specially formulated multi-vitamins with high antioxidant content, high quality omega 3 fish oil supplements, minerals, and specific bionutraceuticals compounded on the basis of cellular regeneration.

4. *Brain Wave Modification and Biofeedback.* In these experimental treatments, children are taught to use calming techniques to control the brainwave patterns that lead to sustained attention or concentration. This technique is rarely, if ever, used in conjunction with MRI information demonstrating the functional areas of the brain that show impairment.

5. *Behavioral Therapy.* A therapist meets regularly with the family and the child to discuss rules, consequences (positive and negative) to promote changes in compliance and follow-through. There has been a great disservice to children with

ADD/ADHD in that the individual, family, and/or group work needed for this population is seen as a "school problem" because the children have difficulty concentrating or learning. At various ages, however, ADD/ADHD and other learning disabilities are encountered everywhere and are not limited to the academic environment. They are neurological disorders that affect the basic skills of social living. The increased risk of depression, anxiety, and other problems in living, make it essential that these children have access to therapy from early on in their development.

Since I have already mentioned specific impairments in the brain, a little anatomy lesson seems to be in order (sorry, but it may help). Look at the brain in the next three diagrams. Notice how it seems all wrinkled and divided by folds and fissures. If we follow some of these large creases, we see that from front to back the brain is divided into two halves or hemispheres that make up the right and the left sides. This part of the brain that you can see is called the cerebrum or cerebral cortex. It is not very thick and covers the rest of the brain like a blanket. Each hemisphere is divided again, by its creases, into lobes or major sections. These sections include the frontal lobes (in the front or anterior region of the brain, again looking down on it, from the nose back); the parietal lobes (behind the frontal lobes proceeding backwards or posterior in direction); and the occipital lobes (behind or posterior to the parietal lobes). On the sides of these hemispheres are the temporal lobes.

The subcortical regions underneath the cortex are the parts of the brain which are only visible in the crossed section drawing. Again, while very complex, we can summarize these parts and collections of parts into two basic areas. Firstly, there is the limbic system, a horseshoe like set of structures that encircles the center of the brain. Secondly, there is the structure in the center of the brain itself that rises up into the horseshow shaped limbic system and is called the brain stem, which includes the reticular activating system (RAS) which provides the brain with a "wake up call" whenever new information is arriving from other parts of the body. At the back of the brain, also located underneath the cortex is the cerebellum. This structure has to do with balance and the integration of data from other parts of the brain, as well as other functions. Although the brain has many other parts, it is important to know that for our purposes the following are most relevant.

When we talk about the structure of the brain we can say:

1. The cortex deals with thinking and the integration of perception and sensory input. Sensory integration and motor output is localized in the back half of the cortex. What we call thinking occurs in the front part of the cortex and includes assessment, delay, integration, judgment and the ability to profit from experience, which implies memory.
2. The brain stem, which is the oldest part of the brain developmentally, has to do with arousal and the autonomic nervous system, which controls breathing and heart-rate, etc. without conscious awareness.
3. The limbic system, which is also an older portion of the brain from a

developmental standpoint, has to do with feelings and memory.

When we talk about the functioning of the brain we can say:

1. The brain, like every other organ and organ system, consists of specialized cells. The cells in the brain are called neurons of which there are many types. At this level of brain function, it is instructive to talk about the chemical and electrical aspects of the brain. The brain chemicals that we are concerned with are called neurotransmitters. Many of them have been reported in the press, and most psychotropic drugs work in large part by altering the levels of these chemicals. For example, serotonin is linked with mood disorders, and most modern anti-depressants work by raising the brain's level of serotonin.
2. Information travels around the brain by electrical impulses and chemical reactions, as it does in the rest of your body. When we think about the ways in which medications work in the brain we are talking about the effect such compounds have on these electro-chemical processes.

A Brief Note on Adult ADHD

Attention Deficit Hyperactivity Disorder (ADHD) in children frequently persists into adolescence and adulthood. Although it has been estimated that approximately 10% of school-aged children in the United States meet the criteria for ADHD, follow-up studies suggest that 30% to 60% of these childhood ADHD cases persist into adulthood. In other words, potentially 6 to 10 million adults in this country are affected by ADHD, with only about 2 million adults receiving prescriptions for ADHD drugs, and as many as 7 million adults not receiving any medication at all. Adult ADHD clearly remains under-diagnosed and under-treated.

Since the core symptoms of ADHD (hyperactivity, impulsivity, and inattention) do not decline significantly with age, adults with ADHD experience functional impairments academically, professionally and in social and emotional relationships. They are prone to explosive moods and antisocial behavior and are more likely to abuse drugs and alcohol, be arrested, be involved in traffic violations and accidents, and have an increased risk of developing comorbid diseases such as depression, anxiety, or bipolar disorder.

Adult ADHD has a substantial economic impact as well. Adults with the disorder have much lower graduation rates, educational attainments in general, and household income, while suffering increased health care costs and health care system utilization rates.

Medications for the treatment of childhood ADHD can also decrease impairment and increase functioning in adults. As with children, stimulant therapy is considered the primary mode of treatment. Prescribing physicians still disagree on their preference for immediate release versus long-acting stimulants. One problem with immediate release formulations is that they often require multiple dosing during the day and because adults with ADHD tend to be forgetful and disorganized, there has been an impetus to develop once-daily long-acting formulations of stimulant medications during treatment of ADHD.

There has also been an interest in incorporating certain nutritional supplements in the treatment regimens of adults with ADD/ADHD as evidence supporting their use continues to mount. Such nutritional compounds include pharmaceutical grade B vitamins, choline, 5-HTP, cellular bionutraceuticals and very promising Omega 3 fatty acids and fish oil. In conjunction with a healthy diet and daily exercise routine these agents alone or combined with conventional therapies play an important role in the management of adults with ADD/ADHD.

Chapter3

Memory – Getting Sharp and Staying Sharp

It's all About Memory, Mostly

Memory is not just a single concept; it embraces a complex collection of ideas that mental health experts have about the brain and how it functions. It is a system that depends on several areas of the brain and their interrelationships. This series of structures can be seen as a network.

Clinicians talk about three different types of memory within the network – long-term, short-term, and immediate memory. The diagram below represents the connections between memory systems. The goal of our memory system is to get information from Short to Long-Term Memory for storage.

The first level of memory, called Immediate Memory (or the ability to take in sensory data and register or encode it) is placed on the outside of the diagram above. This is because the vast majority of sensory information is not stored in long-term memory. After you have touched a hot stove, you instantly recognize the sensory data of intense heat that burns the skin. You do not have to access that sense memory every time you come near a hot stove. Instead you use a second process called short-term memory to remember not to touch the hot stove while you are cooking, then it's gone. We literally complete thousands of tasks everyday with the combination of sensory and short-term memory.

At the level of Short-Term Memory (STM), the brain takes some of this immediate memory, screens, selects it as relevant, and tells us to attend to it, such as the hot stove. It only lasts from several to thirty seconds, because it only takes moments to realize how hot the stove is. Because of its' short duration of holding items for use and its finite limit of memory space, STM is in a constant state of flux. The finite limit is that STM can hold/use 5-9 items at a time. The second function of STM is to begin the process of "encoding". Encoding involves preparing information for long-term storage. Short-term memory can be encoded in auditory, visual, and sensory modes, like the sound of words or a scene of some event. If we make an effort to repeat or link such data with other associations (e.g. the process of rehearsal), it may stay in our memory longer but takes up more of that precious and limited space of 5-9 items.

In addition, how you encode information often affects its storage and recall. Within your Short-Term Memory and helping to make the bridge to Long-Term Memory is Working Memory. Working Memory refers to holding information in your mind and working on it in some way. This attention is called rehearsal. Thus, over time, such processes help us to sort out, reorganize and set things into a context, which requires the use of speech or images to function in the day-to-day world. Hence the name Working Memory.

Let's Try an Experiment: Memory Methods and Techniques

If you try to remember a phone number - 123 456 7890 - that is 10 items. However, there are several ways to remember these numbers. I already mentioned one: rehearsal. You could repeat this number over and over until you can recall it. It may take 10 or 15 repetitions before you can remember the number easily. Or, you could try a strategy called "chunking" or grouping the numbers so that they take up less space in STM for encoding. For example, 123 is the area code, 456 is the exchange, and 7890 is the last for digits. If you try to remember the numbers by this method you have, in effect reduced 10 bits of information to 3. You could even reduce it to one piece of information if you happen to notice that the numbers are all in a sequence from 1 to 10. That is "chunking" the data. You will easily remember this number now. The mental gymnastics associated with rehearsal and chunking are both examples of Working Memory in action.

Your Long-Term Memory and How It Works

Long-term memory refers to anything stored for at least thirty seconds, and can remain for an unlimited duration. Each type of memory is associated with a different brain region and impairment in any one area will affect that particular type of memory storage and retrieval.

Long-Term Memory has two main divisions:

> Declarative memory - also called Explicit Memory because it consists of memories for facts or events such as birthdays, phone numbers and the names of your children

> Non-declarative memory - otherwise known as Implicit Memory because it consists of routines such as procedures as well as sensory, reflexive, and emotional responses.

Your brain does a marvelous job of keeping these memories separate and distinct, but we are also able to merge explicit and implicit memories as well. You may remember times where the family was together for a special day such as a holiday gathering. The event (declarative/explicit) will be remembered more robustly with other sensory memory information and emotional response memory (non-declarative/implicit) such as the smells of the meal, the laughter shared, or the happiness you felt at the time.

If My Brain Is So Good At All Of These Processes, Then Why Can't I Remember?

As it so happens, although parts of your brain work together to make memories more robust, they can and do work independently as well. For example, many individuals with Alzheimer's are at greater risk in their own homes when they remember how to turn on the stove and even drive a car. This is referred to as procedural memory or remembering how to do a task. However, they do not have the declarative memory capacity to remember why and/or when they turned on the stove or where they were going in the car. Hence, the memory for the procedure can be dangerous for them without the other memory systems helping to guide its use.

So what is actually happening when you can't find your car keys or remember someone's name or what you came upstairs for? Here are some of the causes for these types of memory failure:

Reason 1: Memory not stored/encoded. Not deemed important enough to activate the encoding system.

Reason 2: Disorganization: Organization/sorting of the material to be remembered is poor.

Reason 3: Distraction. Other items occupy the space in Short-Term Memory that dislodges the information from the above questions.

Reason 4: Brain Damage. One or more systems or structures in the brain is malfunctioning due to some illness or damage.

Reason 5: A combination of two or more of the above factors.

The reason we forget events like this is largely due to distraction combined with another interfering issue. Distraction interferes with Immediate, Short-Term and Long-Term memory. To hold a piece of information in memory long enough to use it, it must be kept relevant and fresh. When we lose our car keys, forget a name or phone number, forget what we were looking for upstairs, we have not refreshed the memory well enough to use it. You weren't trying to remember it forever, just until you needed it.

Emotions and their impact on memory

Emotions further complicate Working Memory, Encoding, and Long-Term Memory. When you can't remember where your keys are you become frustrated, angry and fearful. These emotions interfere with memory. Individuals with moderate to severe dementia often cannot retrace the events that made them so frustrated or fearful. For those experiencing memory problems, questions become more frequent which produces still more anxiety further interrupting their ability to remember or function in general.

Structural damage to the brain can significantly interact with emotional and, by extension, memory functioning. If one's frontal lobe is damaged, "executive" skills such as attention, planning, judgment, delay, various kinds of awareness, insight and flexibility, as well as the feelings of rage or apathy can change dramatically. Damage to the right side of the brain during a stroke can significantly impact emotional functioning and may well interfere with memories associated with emotion.

What Can I Do To Help My Memory?

It is important to bear in mind that a loss of memory is not remediated in a day. If you have been steadily neglecting to keep your memory capabilities sharp, it will take time to reengage the systems you need and establish both new habits and procedures for remembering.

Organizing Your Memories

Exercise 1:

Organizing Memory

Step 1.	Put together a list of needed information.
Step 2.	Put the information on index cards.
Step 3.	Rehearse and develop chunking strategies.
Example:	My daughter Bonnie lives at 410 Peachtree Way.
	Her number is 123 456 7890.
	Useable/Meaningful chunks:
	Bonnie 410 Peachtree (3 chunks)
	123 456 7890 (3 chunks)

Exercise 2:

Make a Memory Book

Step 1:	Collect pictures, numbers, important dates, and information.
Step 2:	Place pictures, names, birthdates, and important information on one page of the book. Buy a large size book (81/2 x 11), it is easier to organize. Use rubber cement or other sticky substance so that you can easily remove, reorganize, or change the layout of the page.
Step 3:	Make regular updates to the book.
Step 4:	Keep the book with you at all times if possible.

Improving Problems with Attention

Exercise 1:

Goal: Increasing Attention Span

Step 1: Limit distractions. Turn off the television, radio, bright lights, and use filters such as softer lighting, sound machines/white noise machines.

Step 2: Pick a particular spot for work, reading, or hobbies requiring sustained attention.

Step 3: Make this area distraction free. Choose a well-lit, uncluttered space without a television or radio nearby

Step 4: Make it manageable. Limit the amount of work placed in this area at one time.

Step 5: Make it routine. Set the time and task to be accomplished on a schedule. If you know how long or how much you have to do, it will be easier to maintain attention.

Step 6: Clear the area of all clutter after task completion. Throw out garbage, junk mail, old newspapers etc. to keep the area useable.

Exercise 2:

Goal: Increasing the ability to selectively attend to the desired information and filter out distractions to minimize the risk of interference.

Step 1: Time yourself as you complete a short maze, crossword or search-a-word puzzle with the radio/television on and the volume loud. This will determine your ability to filter out distracting information from the task at hand or selectively attend to the task of interest.

Step 2: Time yourself without the distractions while you complete a similar length task. As your selective attention improves, the time with and without distraction should begin to equalize (even though you will most likely remain somewhat slower on the distraction task).

Training Your Ability to Recall

Exercise 1: **Recognition Recall**

Goal: Identify learned material from sense information (auditory/visual/tactile)

Step 1:	Make a list of information to recall (no greater than 9 items).
Step 2:	Rehearse 5 times.
Step 3:	Have a partner make up a list of 11 more items that were not on the original list for a grand total of 20 items.
Step 4:	Have a partner quiz you on the original list of items asking whether or not an item was on the list.

Exercise 2: Recognition Recall

Goal: Envisioning strategies to use other areas of memory (visual and spatial) to help with recognition and recall.

Step 1:	Construct a Spider Map. A Spider Map is a series of interconnected balloons with information inside often leading to a point or tracing some logical memory process (see diagram below).
Step 2:	Trace lines in spider map and repeat each step aloud.
Step 3:	Spider maps may be used to remediate wandering behavior or improve directional sense. It often helps to walk the route for wandering behavior and repeat the directions repeatedly as the "wanderer" reads a copy of the spider map.

Other ideas to improve recognition
Use external aids and visual reminders.
Create a Diary
Post-it notes

Exercise 3: Associative/Cued Recall

Goal - Develop category references to the stored information to make storage and retrieval of information more efficient.

Step 1:	Make a list of items that need to be recalled.
Step 2:	Pegging – use rhyming words or objects to help with recall of details.
Step 3:	Use concrete associations. Tony = Baloney; Michael = Motorcycle.
Step 4:	Use associations that make sense to you. If you have a special name

or detail for a certain person or item, use it. You'll remember it with far greater frequency.

Step 5:   Pick unusual but obvious facts and/or features to remember. The doctor was tall/short/round etc. He was the foot doctor or the head doctor (shrink). Hey, if it helps you remember, no one should be offended.

Step 6:   Situational cues. How do you know this person? For example, that is Mary. She is my nurse. She works on the 2nd shift. Some older adults learn and remember their nurses by the days they work at the facility (Sally Saturday and Terry Tuesday).

Exercise 3:   Free Recall

Goal- Recall information without the use of specifically designed encoding/storage cues.

Step 1:   Generate a list of information.

Step 2:   Visualization – creating images of the object to be remembered

Step 3:   Use all the senses you can – tactile, olfactory, auditory, visual, ustatory, and kinesthetic information to make the image stronger.

Step 4:   Make up stories that are sense related and contain the needed information.

Step 5:   Write the story. (Alternate learning pathway)

Step 6:   Make the story into a ballad and sing it. (Alternate learning pathway)

Additional Memory Exercises

Facial Recognition

Step 1:   Look clearly at the person

Step 2:   Write down details about their appearance

Step 3:   Rhyme or develop simple means for memorizing names

Step 4:   Repeat the list and test yourself once every 20 minutes for 1 hour to solidify the memory and the recall ability

List Recall

Step 1:   Make up a list of 9 items

Step 2:   Write the list

Step 3:   Read the list

Step 4:   Sing the list

Step 5:   Incorporate sensory information into the memory of the list (colors, shapes, sounds, tastes, smells)

Step 6:   Incorporate active movement into the words on the list to be remembered.
   a.   Can you draw the object?
   b.   Can you act out the object (like charades)?
   c.   Can you move to where the object is located?

Step 7:   Reorder the list visually
   a.   Put the words in a tic-tac-toe board frame or grid

   •   Write the words down on a sheet of paper and cut them into strips of paper with one object to be remembered per strip
   •   Draw a tic-tac-toe board on a separate sheet of paper.
      Place them on the tic-tac-toe board and try to remember where they were on the page.
      Then place the items randomly and repeat trying to remember the words and their location on the page.

Step 8:   Personalize the list
   a. Make up sentences that link the object with you personally
   •   My daughter's name is Doris
   •   I must got to the store and buy milk

Step 9:   Recall the list

Word Finding

Step 1:   Make a list of 9 words

Step 2:   Across from each word write 3 words with similar meanings

Step 3:	Use a thesaurus to check for accuracy
Step 4:	Recall the list
Step 5:	Recall the three synonyms for each word
Step 6:	Recall the original list word and the three synonyms. Do this for all 9 words, one at a time
Step 7:	Recall the entire original list of all 9 words

Name Finding

Step 1:	Write a list of 9 important names to remember
Step 2:	Across from each name write 3 important details about that person
Step 3:	If possible, include a picture of the person to remember
Step 4:	Recall the list of names
Step 5:	Recall all the details about the named person
Step 6:	Recall the listed name of the person with the details. Do this for all 9 names, one at a time
Step 7:	Recall the entire list of names

Visual Communication Board (particularly useful when speech dysfunction is present)

Step 1:	Clip pictures of items from magazines or newspapers
Step 2:	Make a collage of these items with the word or phrase attached to them
Step 3:	Use to communicate by pointing to the items or words, but also try to say the names of the items while pointing

Long-Term Memory and Associative Reasoning (not simple recall)

The "Proverbs Test" is a useful measure of recalling prior learned material for some other purpose than simple recall. This "Test" measures and increases the ability to reason using indirect information. By using "old sayings" that we can recall or have heard before, we learn to infer meanings, improve recall, and use verbal problem solving skills as well as our memory

Step 1:   Read each of the following proverbs and explain their meaning:

a. Where there is a will there is a way.

_____

_____

a. Rome was not built in a day.

_____

_____

_____

a. When the cat's away, the mice will play.

_____

_____

_____

Chapter 4

Breaking Bad Habits

Before you start learning about the different ways to enhance your memory skills and cognitive abilities, let's first take a look at areas in which you should STOP doing some things. These are what I call "The Seven Deadly Sins of Intellectual Decline." They are ALL avoidable. They are all things you CAN change, and there is the added benefit of improving your overall health, longevity, and quality of life as well.

1)   Obesity/poor nutrition

2)   Smoking

3)   Alcohol overuse

4)   Inadequate exercise (regardless of one's physical condition)

5)   Using the wrong treatments, e.g. too few, too many, too much or too little vitamin, mineral and/or herbal supplements or unknowingly taking cognition-interfering pharmaceuticals prescribed by your physician to treat a variety of common illnesses (see Chapter 5)

6)   Mental junk food

7)   Emotional junk food

You probably already know that a healthy overall lifestyle improves your physical well being, but did you know it may also help keep your brain healthy as well?

Of course, age is the most critical factor in the development of Alzheimer's and other memory related diseases. Biological and genetic factors also play a role. Although you really do not have much control over any of those variables, you DO have control over "The Seven Deadly Sins of Intellectual Decline." Let's first review them in somewhat greater detail:

Obesity/Poor Nutrition: Your Head and Your Heart

So what does my waist size have to do with my IQ? The short answer is a lot! According to the Alzheimer's Association (2004), "what's good for the heart is good for the brain." That makes perfect sense when you take into consideration that heart disease, high blood pressure (hypertension), stroke, obesity and diabetes are all risk factors for dementia. A Swedish study found that men whose Body Mass Index (BMI) is 30 or higher have a whopping 154 percent greater risk for dementia (The healthy range for BMI for men is between 18.5 and 24.9.)! At the beginning of Chapter 8 I will tell you how to calculate your BMI. If you are overweight, seek consultation from your physician about the advisability of a structured weight-loss program. Many people mistakenly believe that if they are overweight they are at least getting adequate nutrition from their meals. The truth is, however, that many obese individuals overeat on "empty" (i.e., non-nutritious) calories and are actually seriously malnourished. So much for the "Twinkie Diet."

Furthermore, it has been estimated that most people would benefit from eating only 80 percent of what they ordinarily consume at every meal (mayoclinic.com 10/27/03). In fact, new anti-aging research stipulates that one of the key factors in increasing longevity is to work at developing a lean body to the point of becoming 5% underweight. Accomplishing this will not only ameliorate many chronic conditions suffered by people who are overweight, but will also prolong your life by turning back your biological clock and dramatically reducing risk factors for the degenerative diseases of aging.

Consider what weight-loss program or approach may best work for you via consultation with a psychologist and/or registered dietician who specializes in weight-loss and weight-management. People are overweight for a variety or reasons and, conversely, can lose weight in a variety of ways. Not every method yields the same result, however, so getting a proper consultation at the onset of a weight-loss program rather than starting on your own may keep you from frustrating false starts, wasted effort, and malnutrition. Care must also be taken to avoid fad diets. The latest food crazes are often designed for short-term benefits and can often actually cause HARM to your overall physical health and, by extension, your cognitive and emotional health as well.

In the meantime, make sure you eat plenty of antioxidant rich foods. These foods include dark fruits and vegetables (see Chapter 7 for more on healthy eating and losing weight), or take a supplement rated highly as an antioxidant. Watch what you eat to ensure your cholesterol levels are where they should be to help avoid increased risk of heart disease and stroke.

Do You Smoke?

If your answer is yes, STOP! It causes you and everyone around you harm. In fact, smoking reduces the amount of oxygen that your brain gets, thus decreasing its ability to function at its fullest. In addition to being a key risk factor for cancer, it also increases risk for memory impairing strokes and heart disease. Recent research also suggests that children of mothers who smoked during pregnancy had a much higher risk of developing Attention Deficit Hyperactivity Disorder (ADHD), an all too common neurological disorder which I've already noted adversely affects concentration and attention, increases physical aggression, and often hinders social and academic development.

Just as dieting is easier said than done, I know it can be difficult to stop smoking and even more difficult to *stay* smoke free. As with weight loss, our best advice is to learn more about which smoking-cessation program or approach is likely to work best for you via consultation with a medical or health psychologist who specializes in smoking-cessation. For more details and specifics, please see the Resource section at the end of this book for programs to help you stop smoking.

Alcohol Overuse

Like smoking, alcohol intoxication does much to dull one's cognitive abilities. There are also other risks such as falling, automobile accidents, and citations for Driving Under the Influence (DUI) or Driving While Intoxicated (DWI). Besides, hangovers are unpleasant, and never worth the fun you thought you had the night before, dancing around with that lampshade on your head. Alcohol also interferes with the action and/or absorption of pharmaceuticals or nutraceuticals you may be taking which can cause dehydration, liver and/or kidney problems, and various other avoidable ills, even death.

Korsakoff's disease, Wernikie-Korsakoff's disease or Wernikie's encephalapathy results from long-term alcohol use in tandem with Vitamin B-1 (thiamine) deficiency. These conspire to produce significant memory loss, which may be reversed at least in part through sobriety, proper diet, and nutritional therapy.

Some recent research findings may have confused the issue regarding the effect of alcohol on overall health. That is, alcohol can actually raise blood levels of HDL, or "good" cholesterol, and thus help in preventing atherosclerosis or hardening of the arteries, but only if consumed in moderation. This research notes that "moderate" alcohol intake means no more than one "drink" per day for women and two for men. A "drink" is defined as 12 ounces of beer, 3 to 4 ounces of wine, or 1.5 ounces of 80-proof spirits. A study published in 2003 in the *Journal of the American Medical Association* found that subjects over 65 who had one drink a day had half the risk of Alzheimer's compared to non-drinkers. However, those who were heavy drinkers had a 22% *higher* risk than nondrinkers did. While no healthcare professional in their right mind is going to "prescribe" drinking alcohol, especially if you're on medication, it does appear that moderate use may lower cholesterol levels as well as delay the onset of Alzheimer's –of course, so may a number of other more nutritious options!

Alcohol addiction is a separate problem unto itself, which in addition to all of the problems associated with overuse, can lead to financial, employment, familial, social, emotional, psychological and criminal difficulties as well. Again, our best advice is to seek a consultation with a mental health professional that specializes in alcohol addiction or abuse in order to get potentially life saving treatment. For more details and specifics, I have listed some appropriate websites and programs at the end of this book.

Inadequate Exercise (Regardless of one's physical condition!)

As an ode to the proverbial Couch Potato, I have heard just about every excuse in the book to NOT exercise – it's too hot/it's too cold, it's too sunny/it's too dark, I'm too tired/I'm too busy, I have to work/I'm on vacation – the list is endless. It is too bad we cannot burn enough calories, build muscle, or get much aerobic benefit from coming up with creative excuses for NOT exercising.

Many of us consider exercise an all-or-none proposition. That is, we often do not think that it is worth it to put on some comfortable shoes and just walk or jog around the block – too much hassle for too little assumed benefit. So instead, we do nothing! Not very logical, but all too common.

Exercise need not involve running marathons or bench-pressing 300 pounds. What exercise needs to be is tailored to your current ability, perhaps with a goal in mind to help with motivation, and regularly engaged in. Yes, it can be that simple. Can't jog around the block? OK, try walking around it. Can't do that? OK, walk halfway. Can't touch your toes when standing? OK, try it while sitting or touch your knees while standing. As little as 20 to 30 minutes of walking, swimming, or biking per day can be quite helpful, and as few as 8 minutes of resistance exercises twice a week can greatly increase strength, balance and bone health while decreasing the risk of falling, one of the major causes of fragility fractures in the elderly.

Exercise is mentally important as it helps to increase and/or maintain good blood flow to the brain, and studies also indicate that it can actually encourage the growth of new brain cells (mayoclinic.com 10/27/03). It also helps decrease heart disease, stroke and diabetes risk – which is good for your cognitive functioning as well! (See chapter 8 for more on developing a healthy exercise plan suited to your needs and abilities.)

Using The Wrong Treatments

Just like the old adage that no good deed goes unpunished, many of us conscientiously working to regain or maintain our health only *further impair our memories!* For example, using multiple sub-specialty physicians who are not in frequent communication with each other can result in uncoordinated medicating that can lead to memory loss – as well as other possible problems. The help of an appropriate clinical case manager (often a primary care physician or a nurse practitioner) to coordinate medical care and the proper use of multiple medications (sometimes referred to as "poly-pharmacy") can be critically helpful.

Alternatively, in our zeal to be optimally healthy, we may wind-up wastefully spending great amounts of money on vitamins, minerals, and other nutritional supplements that are poorly absorbed and utilized by our bodies. On the other hand, we may be putting ourselves at risk for inadvertently overdosing on fat-soluble vitamins (like vitamins A, D, E or K) that we do not readily metabolize and run the risk of neurological problems like hypervitaminosis and liver toxicity. Even if you have carefully researched the amounts you should be taking, if the supplements are not pharmaceutical grade (i.e. "nutraceuticals"), there is no way of knowing how many milligrams you're actually absorbing.

The literature can also be incredibly confusing concerning the use and misuse of vitamins, minerals, herbs, over the counter preparations, even prescription medications. Upcoming chapters will provide you with the latest information to help in reconciling the confusing and seemingly mixed signals that too often appear in the popular press and media.

Mental Junk Food

In this chapter, we have covered issues related to poor bodily nutrition but, as clinical psychologists, I can tell you that there is also such a thing as "mental junk food" that is likewise filled with empty cognitive calories. That is, a steady diet of junk television does little to stimulate your mind or your spirit. What qualifies as mental junk food? Basically, anything that fills you up but has little redeeming value. Television that passes the time but doesn't impress, inspire, teach or stimulate you to think. Consider the difference in watching an hour's worth of Jerry Springer versus PBS' Frontline or 60 Minutes. Frankly I'd prefer 90 minutes in a theater watching a Buster Keaton revival to watching a Dodge ball championship anytime.

We all know that quality entertainment is in the eye and ear of the beholder, but good is good and, frankly, trash is trash. A bad television show or movie now and then will not make you a dolt – just like the occasional candy bar or piece of cake will not kill you, but a steady media diet of trash does not prep you for the Mental Olympics either. The choice is yours.

Emotional Junk Food

Similar to mental junk food, emotional junk food refers to something you may spend a lot of time and emotional effort with that leaves you feeling unsatisfied not long thereafter. This could be a one-sided friendship where you do most of the supporting and receive little when you are in need. Alternatively, constantly being used and unappreciated in a friendship or supposedly loving relationship. There are a variety of reasons why one maintains such negative relationships. A mental health professional can help you sort through such complicated issues, without bias, and with your best interests in mind. In the meantime, if this area concerns you, look at Chapter 9 for some tips and actionable ideas to consider.

Next Step

In summary, it is critically important to do all that you can to minimize or, even better, eliminate as many of these bad habits as possible. Before you can begin to build or maintain your brainpower, you will first have to do some repairs to your unhealthy habits. Doing so may not be easy, but you will experience a double benefit (both cognitively and physically) when you succeed.

Chapter 5

Supplements and Nutraceuticals

As noted in the previous chapter, some things considered good for us at one point in time are later found to not be as helpful as first thought, if not outright dangerous. I also explained the processes of scientific research methodology and the problems with the popular media rarely noting the limitations of "important" new studies.

Now, there are a number of vitamins (e.g. B complex and E), Anti-oxidants (e.g. ALA, Coenzyme Q_{10}, etc.), Amino Acids, Minerals, Phytomedicinals (e.g. Ginkgo Biloba), and "Nutraceuticals" (pharmaceutical-grade nutrient combinations like Phyto-Vite) available that are all considered potentially helpful for memory and cognitive functioning. For the present chapter I have compiled and synthesized currently available literature to help you make sense and, more importantly, proper use of non-prescription supplements. You will also want to consider this chapter in the context of Chapter 8 and how to structure your diet to gain optimal nutrition.

The following is a handy listing of what is generally or widely accepted as reliable and scientifically (evidence-based) information;*

Substance	Benefits	Strength of Evidence	Therapeutic Daily Amount	Side effects/ contraindication
Acetyl-carnitine	"conditionally essential nutrient"	+	250 mg – 1500 mg/d	Rare side effects include increased appetite, nausea, headache, agitation. People with kidney and liver disease should not take it without a physician's supervision
	-improvement of overall cognitive functioning	+ +	most studies suggest 500-1000 mg/d	
	-delay in onset of age related cognitive decline	+		
	-delay in progression of Alzheimer's Disease	+ +		

Alpha-lipoic acid (ALA)	-potent antioxidant	+ + +	50 mg/d	Not known
	-suspected to assist in memory maintenance	0/ +	up to 600 mg/d for diabetic neuropathy	
	-enhances glucose uptake in non-insulin dependent diabetes	+ +	maximum safe level up to 1800 mg/d	
	-improves diabetic neuropathy	+		
B Vitamins	stimulate memory, helpful in stress and management of depression			None, however pregnant women need to take it with a physician's supervision
	improve reaction time in children			
Thiamine – B₁	enhances neuro-transmission from brain to spinal chord	+ +	RDA 1.4 mg/d Range 1.4-100 mg	
Riboflavin – B₂	-may be useful in people with burns, chronic diarrhea, liver disease aid cancer	+/+ +	RDA 1.3 mg/d Range 25-100 mg Max safe level 280 mg	Interferes with certain medications (phenothiazines, tricyclic antidepressants, probenecid)
	-may decrease frequency of migraines	+/+ +		
Niacin – B3	-vital for energy release in tissues	+ +	50-100 mg/d for lowering cholesterol up to 1500 mg/d	Flushing (temporary) people with bleeding problems, diabetes, gout, glaucoma, liver disease or ulcers need to consult physician before use
	-helps maintain healthy nervous, digestive system	+ +		

	-improves cholesterol	+ + +		
Pyridoxine – B_6	-essential for healthy nervous system, metabolism of fats, proteins and carbohydrates	+ + +	50-100 mg/d safe up to 200 mg/d	-doses higher then 200 mg/d may lead to nerve damage in the long term
	-helpful in moral control (PMS, depression)	+		-it may decrease effectiveness of L-dopa used to treat Parkinson's disease
	-stress management	+		
Folic Acid – B_9	-reduction of neural tube defects (Spina Bifida) and other birth defects	+ + +	400-800 mcg/d	Very high doses may trigger seizures in people with epilepsy
	-decrease in homocysteine thus lowering risk of stroke and heart attack as well as Alzheimer's disease	+ +		
Cyanocobalamin – B_{12}	-supplementation may improve cognitive function in the elderly	+ +	500-1000 mcg/d RDA 2.4 mcg/d	No side effects from oral forms, but allergic reactions to injectable B12 reported but are rare
		+ +	Maximum safe level 3000 mcg/d	
	-improvement of fatigue			

Choline	-improvement of short term memory - integral part of neurotransmitter acetylcholine	+ +	400 mg/d for women 550 mg/d for men (3.5 g = maximum safe level)	None in recommended doses; abdominal pain, nausea, diarrhea when recommended dose is exceeded
Coenzyme Q_{10}	Powerful antioxidant -prevents skin aging -slows progression of Parkinson's disease -improves congestive heart failure -may be of benefit in AIDS, angina, cancer, diabetes, muscular dystrophy and obesity	+ + + + + + + + +	30-300 mg/d as high as 1200 mg/d for Parkinson's disease	Both may interact positively or negatively with many prescription drugs. Consult your physician if you are currently taking medication.
Vitamin E**	Potent antioxidant -slows rate of mental decline -lowers risk of Alzheimer's disease -may boost immune system -improves reproduction health in women	+ + + + + + + +	400-1200 IU/d best obtained from natural supplements containing d-alphatocopherol US RDA = 8mg (12 IU) for women 10 mg (15 IU) for men European RDA = 15 mg (22IU) maximum safe level 400-800 IU	Vit E should not be taken with supplements or medications which affect clotting (i.e. large doses of aspirin or the blood thinning drug warfarin (genre name) as it may cause further blood thinning. Avoid taking 72 hours before elective surgery.
Omega-3 Fatty Acids and fish oil	-lowers cardiovascular risk	+	1000-3000 mg/d Most supplements contain only 18% EPA and 12% DHA (newly available	If doses greater than 3000 mg taken by patients on prescription medications, consult physician as there may be nutrient/drug

Comprised of: (1) DHA (docosahexanoic acid) (2) EPA (eicosa-pentaenoic acid)	-decrease triglyceride levels -lower blood pressure -reduce serum homosystems -thin blood -help in inflammatory arthritis -improve depression -slow down cognitive decline of aging -help retard progression of Alzheimer's	+ + + + + + + + + + + + + +	nutraceutical delivers 88% DHA and 60% EFA)	interactions, major side-effect is a fishy taste
Ginkgo Biloba	-antioxidant -inhibits platelet aggregation -protects against cardiovascular diseases -supports brain functioning via improved circulation	+ + + + + + +	40-60 mg 3x day (not to exceed 300 mg/d) of standardized extract (24% flavoglycosies) must not have more than 5 parts per million of alkylphenols (toxic compounds found in leaves)	Large doses may lead to headaches, dizziness, and bleeding, especially if also taking aspirin or a blood thinning medication; consult physician before use
Griffonia Simplicifolia	-rich source of 5-HTP (5-hydroxytryptophan, the precursor of neurotransmitter serotonin) - increases CNS synthesis of serotonin - helps in treatment of depression - promotes early feeling of satiety, helps suppress	+++ ++ ++ ++ ++	From 150-600 mg three times a day	Don't combine with SSRI's without a physician's supervision; those with kidney and/or liver disease should only take under a physician's supervision

	emotional eating			
	- helps reduce migraine headaches	+		
	- helps reduce symptoms of fibromyalgia	++		
	- reduces sleep latency time and helps alleviate some types of insomnia	++		
SAM e	-potent chondroprotective agent (slows down progression of arthritis) -helps in treatment of depression -helps in managing pain associated with fibromyalgia	+	400 mg 3-4 times a day	No known side effects

Human Growth Hormone	-enhances energy -improves immune system -improves appearance of skin	+ + +	Recommended for individuals with documented deficiency -low dose, high frequency regimens twice daily	None in small doses, fluid retention and joint pain in large doses.

	-improves mood	+		
	-improves sleep	+		
	-increases lean body mass	+		
	-decreases body fat	+		

Strength of evidence:

0 no support in the literature
+ anecdotal plus some support in literature
+ + fair-good support in literature
+ + + strong support in literature

* Always check with a healthcare professional BEFORE making any changes in your medication or supplement intake since doses can vary as a function of your age, health condition, other medications being taken, diet restrictions, allergies, etc.

** An additional Note on Vitamin E: although some studies report that vitamin E does not result in better memory or a lower risk of getting Alzheimer's Disease, other more recent studies have found that diets rich in vitamin E may indeed help prevent Alzheimer's.

According to a 2002 study in *The Journal of the American Medical Association*, involving 815 men and women (age 65 and older and without Alzheimer's), those who consumed the largest amounts of vitamin E from the food they ate were far less likely to develop Alzheimer's later on. Whatever role other nutrients in the food besides Vitamin E may have played is not clear.

Another 2002 study in *The Journal of the American Medical Association* found that a dietary intake high in vitamin E lowered the risk of developing Alzheimer's. Lastly, a 1997 study in *The New England Journal of Medicine* reported that very large amounts of vitamin E supplement (1000 IU twice daily) might slow the progress of Alzheimer's. However, I do not recommend such a high daily dose, especially on a "maybe" result.

What Is Vitamin E?

Vitamin E is a fat-soluble vitamin, which exists in eight different forms, each having its own biological activity. In humans, Alphatocopherol is the name of the most active form of vitamin E. Vitamin supplements are usually sold as Alphatocopherol acetate or succinate. The synthetic form labelled "D, L" while the natural form is labelled "D." The synthetic form is only half as active as the natural form (Note: 400 IU's of vitamin E per day—the lowest recommended dose—is the equivalent of about 268 mg of the natural form of E and 180 mg of the synthetic form).

Medication-Nutrient Interactions

Some medications cause depletion in certain nutrients. The net result then is that taking such medications for specific illnesses may inadvertently cause a nutrient depletion that can then negatively affect other aspects of health and wellness, as well as adversely impact your memory and concentration. The following tables will help you understand whether some of the problems you or a loved one are experiencing could actually be the result of a nutritional depletion secondary to medications being taken. As noted before, DO NOT alter the present dose or suddenly stop taking a prescribed medication without first consulting the prescribing physician. If you are concerned about possible side effects and/or drug interactions, you can also contact your pharmacist.

Medication– Nutrient Depletion Tables*

Antacids

Medication	Nutrient Depleted
Aluminum hydroxide	Calcium
Magnesium hydroxide	Phosphorus
Magnesium oxide	
Magnesium sulfate	Potassium
Aluminum hydroxide and magnesium hydroxide	
Aluminum hydroxide and magnesium carbonate	
Aluminum hydroxide and magnesium trisilicate	
Aluminum hydroxide and simethicone	
Sodium Bicarbonate	

Medication– Nutrient Depletion Tables*

Antibiotics

Medication	Nutrient Depleted
Cephalosporins	Bifidium (bifidus)
Fluoroquinolones	Vitamin B1
Macrolides	Vitamin B2
Aminoglycosides	Vitamin B3
	Vitamin B6
	Vitamin B12

	Biotin
	Inositol
	Vitamin K
Tetracyclines, sulfonamides	Calcium – take several hours apart from antibiotic
	Magnesium
	Iron
	Lactobacillus acidophilus, Bifidobacteria
	Bifidium
	Vitamin B1
	Vitamin B2
	Vitamin B3
	Vitamin B6
	Vitamin B12
	Biotin Inositol
	Vitamin K
Neomycin	Beta-carotene
	Iron
	Vitamin A
	Vitamin B12
Co-trimoxazole	Bifidobacteria bifidum (bifidus)
	Lactobacillus acidophilus
	Folic acid
Isoniazid	Vitamin B6
INH	Vitamin B3
	Vitamin D
Rifampin	Vitamin D
Ethambutol	Zinc
	Copper

Medication– Nutrient Depletion Tables*

Anticonvulsants

Medication	Nutrient Depleted
Barbiturates	Vitamin D
	Calcium
	Folic acid
	Vitamin K
Phenytoin	Biotin
	Vitamin D
	Calcium
	Folic acid
	Vitamin K
	Vitamin B12
	Vitamin B1
Carbamazepine	Folic acid
	Vitamin D
	Biotin
Primidone	Folic acid
	Biotin
Valproic acid	Folic acid
	Carnitine

Medication– Nutrient Depletion Tables*

Antidiuretics

Medication	Nutrient Depleted
Sulfonylureas	Coenzyme Q10
Acetohexamide	"
Glyburide	"

Tolazamide	"
Biguanicies	Vitamin B12
Metformin	"

Anti-Inflammatories

Medication	Nutrient Depleted
Salicylates	Vitamin C
Aspirin	Folic Acid
Choline magnesium trisalicylate	Potassium
Choline salicylate	Iron
	Sodium
Salisalate	Folic acid
Nonsteroidal Anti-Inflammatory Agents Ibuprofen, naproxen, sulindac piroxican, dicifenac, diflunisal, etodoiac, fenoprofen, ketoprofen, ketorolac	Folic acid Malatonin
Nonsteroidal Anti-Inflammatory meclofenamate, nabumetone, tolmetic, mefenamic acid, Celecoxib Indomethacin	Folic acid and iron
Corticosteroids	Calcium
Betamethasone, budesonide	Vitamin D
Cortisone, dexamethasone, Flunisolide, fluticasone Hydrocortisone, mometasone, Methylprednisolone	Potassium
	Zinc
Prednisone, prednisolone	Vitamin C
	Magnesium
Triamcinolone	Folic acid
	Selenium

Antivirals

Medication	Nutrient Depleted
Reverse Transriptase Inhibitors	Copper
Didanosine	Zinc
Lamivudine	Vitamin B12
Stavudine	Carnitine
Zalcitabine	
Zidovudine	
Non-Nucleoside	Copper
Delavirdine	Zinc
Nevirapine	Vitamin B12
	Carnitine

Medication– Nutrient Depletion Tables*

Benzodiazepines

Medication	Nutrient Depleted
Diazepam	Melatonin
Alparazolam	

Bronchodilators

Medication	Nutrient Depleted
Theophylline	Vitamin B6

Cardiovascular Medications

Medication	Nutrient Depleted
Vasodilators	Vitamin B6
Hydralzine	Coenzyme Q10
Loop Diuretics	Calcium
Furosemide	Magnesium
Bumetanide	Vitamin B1
Ethcrynic Acid	Vitamin B6
	Vitamin C
	Potassium
	Zinc
Thiazide Diuretics	Magnesium
Hydrochlorothlazide	Potassium
Methyclothiazide	Zinc
Indapamide	Coenzyme Q10
Metolazone	
Potassium-Sparing Diuretics	Calcium
Triamterene	Folic Acid
Hydrocholorthiazide & triamterene	Zinc
	Calcium
	Folic acid
	Zinc
	Vitamin B6
ACE inhibitors	Zinc
Captopril	

Enalopril

Cardiac Glycosides

Digoxin

	Calcium
	Magnesium
	Phosphorus
	Vitamin B1
Beta-blockers	Coenzyme Q10
Propranolol, metoprolol, atenolol, pindolol, acetutolol, betaxolol, bisoprolol, carteolol, carvedilol, esmolol, labetolol, nadolol, sotalol, tirnolol	Melatonin

Medication– Nutrient Depletion Tables*

Cholesterol-Lowering Drugs

Medication	Nutrient Depleted
HMG-CoA Reductase Inhibitors	Coenzyme Q10
Atorvastatin	
Cerivastatin	
Lovastatin	
Fluvastatin	
Pravastatin	
Simvastatin	
Bile Acid Sequestrants	Vitamin A, beta-carotene, vitamin D, vitamin E, vitamin K, vitamin B12, folic acid, iron, calcium, magnesium, phosphorus, zinc
Cholestyramine	
Colestipol	

Medication– Nutrient Depletion Tables*

Electrolyte Replacement

Medication	Nutrient Depleted
Potassium Chloride (Timed Release)	Vitamin B12

Medication– Nutrient Depletion Tables*

Hormones

Oral Contraceptives	Folic acid
	Tyrosine
	Vitamin B2
	Vitamin B6
	Vitamin B12
	Vitamin C
	Magnesium
	Zinc
Estrogen Replacement (ERT) and Hormone Replacement (HRT) Therapies, estrogen, conjugated estrogens, esterified estrogens, raloxifene, and medroxyprogesterone	Vitamin B6
	Magnesium
	Zinc

Anti-Gout Medications

Medication	Nutrient Depleted
Colchicine	Vitamin B12
	Potassium
	Sodium
	Beta-carotene

Medication– Nutrient Depletion Tables*

Laxatives

Medication	Nutrient Depleted
Mineral oil	Vitamin A
	Beta-carotene
	Vitamin D
	Vitamin E
	Vitamin K
	Calcium
Bisacodyl	Potassium

Psychotherapeutic Agents

Medication	Nutrient Depleted
Tricyclic Antidepressants	Vitamin B2
Amitriptyline	Coenzyme Q10
Desipramine	
Nortriptyline	

Doxepin	
Desipramine	
Phenothiazines	Vitamin B2
Chlorpromazine	Coenzyme Q10
Thioridaxine	
Huphenazine	
Butyrophenones	Coenzyme Q10
Haloperidol	

Medication– Nutrient Depletion Tables*

Ulcer Medications

Medication	Nutrient Depleted
H-2 Receptor Antagonists	Vitamin B12
Cimetidine	Folic Acid
Famotindine	Calcium
Nizatadine	Vitamin D
Ranitidine	Iron
	Zinc
Proton Pump Inhibitors	Vitamin B12
Lansoprazole	
Omeprazole	

Miscellaneous

Medication	Nutrient Depleted
Methotrexate	Folic acid
Penicillamine	Vitamin B6
	Magnesium

	Zinc
	Copper
Acetaminophen	Glutathione

* "Drug and Nutrient Interaction Table," from THE REAL VITAMIN AND MINERAL BOOK by Sheri Lieberman and Nancy Bruning, copyright © 1990 by Sheri Lieberman and Nancy Bruning. Used by permission of Avery Publishing, an imprint of Penguin Group (USA) Inc.

A Few Final Words of Advice

Of course, the best way to gain nutritional value is through good foods prepared in a healthy way. However, doing so is not always easy or convenient for many of us. In addition, as noted above, there is a growing body of evidence that the amounts of some nutrients needed for therapeutic or preventive purposes can far exceed what can easily be gained via diet alone, unless you happen to have the capacity of an elephant for leaves, grass, roots, and bark. In such cases, taking supplements may be well advised. If doing so is to be part of your plan, it is also important to know what to look (out) for. The following table offers some final tips that should be of help.

Watch for...	
Seal of Approval	The US Pharmacopoeia Dietary Supplement Verification Program (or USP-DSVP)
What it means:	Verification that the amounts and strengths of the contents are indeed what the label indicates
	Also, the product should dissolve within 30 – 45 minutes in one's stomach
Marketing Gimmicks	Organic or synthetic vitamins make little difference to your body, but a big difference to your pocketbook – with organics costing more. Interestingly, though, synthetic Vitamin K and folic acid are absorbed into your body more efficiently than organically derived forms.
	Unless you have an allergy or sensitivity to wheat, rice, or lactose you need not pay more for allergen-free vitamins.
Interactions	Just because you can buy a supplement over the counter and without a prescription does not mean consulting with a healthcare professional(s) is not necessary; supplements can, on occasion,

adversely interact with other medications and treatments.

Any ill effects	Let your physician know of any adverse health effects and/or you can contact MedWatch (via 800.FDA-1088) www.fda.gov/medwatch/report/consumer/consumer.htm

Chapter 6

Medications and Pharmaceuticals

How Clinical Science Works (And Sometimes Seems Not To)

It seems as if some things considered good for us at one point in time are later found not to be as helpful as first thought – or perhaps even bad for us, and vice-versa. This can be very frustrating, if not frightening, but why is it so?

Essentially, scientific studies are based on hypotheses, which are often nothing more than "educated guesses." By applying the scientific method, we hope to learn more about the accuracy of our best guess. Sometimes, however, the results lead to still more questions than answers.

The scientific process is relatively slow and methodical. Most research starts in the laboratory – perhaps with chemicals and test tubes or computer simulations and models. Then promising avenues may be tested out with laboratory animals whose size, metabolic rate, and relative life span lead to obtaining results much more quickly for starters. This approach is also considered a more ethical method than using human subjects to discover whether a compound may be toxic. Even though humans share a surprising amount in common genetically with other creatures, this does not always mean a hundred percent translation of a finding in lab animals to humans.

Next on the list comes a human epidemiological (or "observational") study. Examples of these include long-term studies that track certain aspects of a group's health and illness patterns over many years. There will likely be comparison or "control" groups with which the focus or at-risk group shares basic similarities (e.g., age, gender, geographic location, ethnic background, type of illness, working conditions, etc.). Such studies have helped us learn that smoking is a cause of lung cancer that heart problems result in part from high cholesterol, and so forth. Of course, we all know about someone who smoked all their lives and never had lung cancer or who "ate like a horse and had a fine ticker." But, while we may be tempted to hope this will be the case for ourselves and our loved ones, statistically it is quite unlikely.

As a final note, I would like to point out a major problem with research reported in the popular media like newspapers, magazines, television, and so on. Usually only bits or "sound-bites" of a study are headlined and any limitations may not make it into the report or article (remember the expression, "the devil is in the details?"). Rather than taking such information at face-value, it may be wiser to talk to your doctor or other trusted healthcare professional to learn if any reported new finding may be relevant or helpful for you.

Medications That May Help with Memory and Cognitive Functioning

The following table contains a list of medications that some studies have considered in the treatment of dementia (Alzheimer's in particular) and other memory problems. Perhaps you have read or heard about some of these. I have listed each substance by its brand and generic name, noting what type of compound category it is, why it is/was considered to be beneficial, clarification as to what it does not do, and a notation if there are any risks or concerns associated with the substance as well.

Medications That May Help with Memory and Cognitive Functioning*

Substance	Category	Benefit(s)	What it does *not* do	*Comments*
Estrogen	Hormone	Mixed results, but some studies show a delay in Alzheimer's onset	Improve memory	Increased risk of breast cancer (especially if taken for dementia in combination with progesterone)
Tacrine (brand name Cognex)	Cholinesterace Inhibitor	Improves impaired language use, reasoning, memory, focused attention	Mixed findings, not a panacea, does not cure/stop progression of memory loss	Associated with liver damage and other side effects. Must be taken 4x/day
Donepexil (Aricept)	Cholinesterace Inhibitor	Decreases mild-to-moderate dementia symptoms		Taken only once/day, no liver risks. Cost for 30, 10 mg tablets = $132
Galantamine (Razadyne formerly known as	Cholinesterace Inhibitor	For mild to moderate Alzheimer's type dementia		Concern with increased risk of death in some

Reminyl)				patients, taken 2/day. Cost for 30, 8 mg tablets = $75
Rivastigmine (Exelon)	Cholinesterace Inhibitor	Helpful for more rapidly progressing disease states, mild to moderate Alzheimer's disease	Not helpful for slower progressing disease states	Therapeutic dose (6 mg/day or more) is associated with increased side- effects, taken 2/day. Cost for 30, 3 mg tablets is about $76
Memantine (Namenda)	NMDA Receptor Antagonist	Slows progression of cognitive problems, helps improve memory functioning, approved for moderate to severe Alzheimer's	Not a cure for memory impairment or more progressive dementias	Promising compound, well tolerated, few side-effects, usually taken 2x/day, not for patients with kidney problems. Cost for 30, 10 mg tables = $68
Ergold Mesylates (Hydergine)	Ergot Alkaloid	Questionable benefit	Questionable benefit	Large number of side-effects, questionable benefit

* Note:Therapy combining a cholinesterace inhibitor and NMDA receptor antagonist may be used by some clinicians throughout some patients, treatment.

Off-Label Use Medications

Some physicians may select the use of other medications not formulated or FDA approved for use in treating memory and cognition, hence the term "off-label." If your physician chooses to do so, be sure you and/or your loved ones understand the rationale behind your doctor's recommendation. The following table lists the most common off-label medications used, along with their medication category, what the intended or original purpose of the medication was, why a physician may consider prescribing it for cognitive symptoms and any associated risks and concerns.

Off-Label Medications

Category	Medication (generic/brand name)	"Original" Benefit(s)	Why use this?	Risks/Concerns
Statins	Atorvastatin/Lipitor	Lowers cholesterol	High cholesterol correlates with many of the causes of progressive dementia, may play a role in slowing the progression of Alzheimer's	Insufficient evidence to recommend for reducing effects of Alzheimer's
	Simvastatin/Zocor			
	Lovastatin/Mevacor			
Calcium Channel Blockers (CCBs)	Verapamil	Various cardiovascular conditions (e.g., high blood pressure, chest pain)	High levels of calcium in the brain correlate with cognitive decline	Long-term uses of CCBs have been associated with cognitive decline
Non-Steroidial Anti-Inflammatory Drugs (NSAIDs)	Ibuprofen/Advil™ & Motrin™	Anti-inflammatory	Inflammation of the brain is associated with memory loss and Alzheimer's	Evidence is not very solid, side-effect risk to gastrointestinal system and kidneys. Data indicate an apparent increase in cardiovascular and cerebrovascular problems for those taking Naproxen
	Indomethacin			
	Naproxen/ Aleve™ &Anaprox™			
	Celecoxib/ Celebrex™	cox-2 inhibitors		

Anti-Parkinson's Disease Medication	Selegiline/Eldepryl	May slow the progression of Alzheimer's from moderate to more severe stages.	Antioxidant and may slow the ongoing loss of brain cells. Selegiline also increases the supply of certain brain chemicals that become diminished in Alzheimer's disease.	Insufficient evidence to recommend
Antibiotics	Chelators (e.g., Clioquinol)	High affinity for zinc and copper ions	Zinc and copper levels may correlate with progressive memory decline	Early stage discovery, needs more research

Medications that May Interfere with Memory and Cognitive Functioning

For certain people, some medications can and do have negative side-effects on memory, concentration, focus, and other cognitive abilities. The following tables will help you understand whether some of the problems you or a loved one is experiencing could actually be the result of medications being taken. Remember, however, DO NOT alter your dose or abruptly stop taking a medication if you have a concern about it without first consulting with your prescribing physician or some other appropriate healthcare professional such as a pharmacist. Lastly, the following list is by no means complete. The intent is to give you something to think about.

Brand Name - *Generic Name*	*Used to Treat/Regulate*
Acthat - corticotrophin	Systemic
Advil/Motrin - ibuprofen	Pain
Aldactazide - spirolactone	Blood pressure (BP)
Aldomet – methyldopa	Blood pressure
Aleve – naproxen	Pain
Amaryl – glimepiride	Diabetes
Ambien – zolpidem	Sleep aide

Ascriptan – aspirin	Pain
Ascendin – amoxapine	Anti-depressant
Ataraz – hydroxyzine HCL	Cold & allergy
Ativan – lorazepam	Tranquilizer/anti-depressant
Atropine – atrophine sulfate	Stomach problems
Aventyl – nortriptylise	Anti-depressant
Axid – mizatidine	Stomach problems
Azmacort - triamcinolone	Systemic
Bayer – aspirin	Pain
Bentyl –dicyclomine HCL	Stomach problems
Benadryl - diphenhydramine	Colds
Buspar – buspirone	Psychiatric tranquilizer
Butisol – butabarbital	Barfiturate
Catapress – clonidine HCL	Heart
Centrax – prazepan	Psychiatric tranquilizer
Chibroxin - norfloxacin	Antibiotic
Chlor-trimetan – chlorpheniramine maleate	Cold & allergy
Ciloxan/Cipro - ciprofloxacin	Antibiotic
Cipro – ciproploxacin	Antibiotic
Clinoril - sulindac	Pain
Clozaril – chlozapine	Anti-psychotic
Compazine - prochlorperazinc	Psychiatric, stomach
Cogentin – benzotropine	Neuropsychiatric
Cortef – hydrocortisone	Systemic
Cortone Accetate – cortisone	Systemic
Corzide – bendroflumethiazide	Blood pressure
Cytovene – ganciclovir	Antibiotic
Dalmane– flurazepam	Neuropsychiatric/tranquilizer
Daypro - oxaprozin	Pain
Decadron – dexamethazone	Systemic

Deltasone – predisone	Systemic
Demadex – torsemide	Blood pressure
Desyrel – trazoclone	Antidepressant
DiaBeta/Micronase – glyburide	Diabetes
Diabinese - chlorpropamide	Diabetes
Dilantin – phenytoin sodium	Neuropsychitric
Dimetane – brumpheniramine maleate	Cold & allergy
Diprolene?Valisone – betamethasone	Systemic
Disalcid - salalate	Pain
Diupres - reserpine	Blood pressure
Diuril – chlorothiazide	Blood pressure
Doan's Pills – magnesium salicodate	Pain
Doriden – glutethimide	Psychiatric
Duract – bromfenac sodium	Pain
Duraquin - quinidine	Heart
Dyazide – thiamterene	Blood pressure
Elavil – amitriptyline	Antidepressant
Enduron – methyelothiazide	Blood pressure
Equanil – meproganate	Neuropsychiatric
Feldene - piroxicam	Pain
Flexiril – cyclobenzaprine	Muscle relaxant
Glucotrol - glipizide	Diabetes
Halcion – thazalam	Neuropsychiatric/tranquilizer
Haldol – haloperidol	Antipsychotic
Hismanal – astemizole	Cold & allergy
Humalog – insulin lispro	Diabetes
Hydropres – resurpine	Blood pressure
Hygoton – chlorthalidone	Blood pressure
Inderal – propranolol	Blood pressure
Indocin - indomethacin	Pain
Insulin –	Diabetes

Kerlone - betaxolol	Blood pressure
Klonopin – clorazapam	Neuropsychiatric
Lanoxicap – digoxim	Heart
Levaquin – levofloxacin	Antibiotic
Levatol – penbutolol	Blood pressure
Librax – chlordiazepovide	Stomach problems
Librium – chlordiazepoxide	Muscle relaxant
Lidocaine	Heart
Lodine - etodolac	Pain
Lomotil – atripane sulfate	Stomach problems
Lopressor – metaprolol	Blood pressure
Lozol – indapamode	Blood pressure
Ludomol – maprotiline	Antidepressant
Luminol sodium-phenobarbital	Barbiturate
Maxquin - lomefloxacin	Antibiotic
Medrol – methylprednisolone	Systemic
Meclomen – meclofenamate sodium	Pain
Mellaril-thioridazine	Antipsychotic
Metahydrin – trichlormethiazide	Blood pressure
Metreton/Pred Forte – prednisolone acetate	Systemic
Miltown-meprobamate	Neurological/tranquilizer
Moduretic – amiloride	Blood pressure
Myidil – triprolidine	Cold & Allergy
Nalfon – fenoprofen calcium	Pain
Navane-thiothixene	Antipsychotic
Nembutol – penobarbital	Neurological
Neurontin - gabapentin	Muscle relaxant
Noctec- chloral hydrate	Tranquilizer
Noludar - methyprylon	Psychiatric
Normdyne- labetalol	Blood pressure

Norpace – disopyramide phosphate	Heart
Ocuflox – oflixacin	Antibiotic
Optimine – azatadine maleate	Cold & Allergy
Orinase – tolbutamide	Diabetes
Orudis - ketoprofen	Pain
Pepcid – famotidine	Stomach
Penetrex - enoxacin	Antibiotics
Prolixin – flutphenazine	Antipsychotic
Prozac – fluoxetine	Antidepressant
Raxar – grepafloxacin	Antibiotic
Regroton – reserpine	Blood pressure
Relafen – nabumetone	Pain
Reserpine	Heart
Restoril – temazepam	Antidepressant
Salutensin – reserpine	Blood pressure
Sectral – acebutolol	Blood pressure
Ser-ap-es - reserpine	Blood pressure
Seldane – terfenadine	Coldl & allergies
Serax – oxazepam	Neuropsychiatric – tranquilizer
Sinequan – doxepin HCL	Antidepressant
Skelaxin – metaxalone	Muscle relaxant
Soma – carisoprodol	Muscle relaxant
Relafen – nabumetone	Pain
Reserpine	Heart
Skelaxin - metaxalone	Muscle relaxant
Soma - carisoprodol	Muscle relaxant
Sonata – zaleplon	Sleep aide
Stelazine – trifluoperazine	Neuropsychiatric/antipsychotic
Surmontil - trimipramine	Antidepressant
Symmetrel – amantadine HCI	Antibiotics
Tagament - cimentidine	Stomach

Talwin – pentazocine/asprin	Pain
Tavist-D – clemastine fumarate	Cold & allergy
Tenex – guanfacine HCI	Heart
Tenoretic – atenolol	Blood pressure
Tenormin – atenolol	Blood pressure
Thorazine – clorazepate	Antipsychotic
Tofranil - imipramine	Antidepressant
Tolectin – tolmetin sodium	Pain
Tolinase – tolazamide	Diabetic
Triavil – amitriptyline/perphenazine	Antidepressant
Trilisate – choline/magnesium salicylate	Pain
Tranxene – clorazepate	Tranquilizer
Urised – methemamine/methylene blue.salol	antibiotic
Valium - diazepam	Anti-anxiety
Visken – pindolol	Blood pressure
Vistaril – hydroxyzine pamoate	Cold & allergy
Voltaren – diclofenac sodium	Pain
Wellbutrin – buproprion HCL	Antidepressant
Xanax – alprazolam	Sleep aide
Zagam - sparfloxacin	Antibiotic
Zantac - ranitidine	Stomach
Zaroxolyn – metolazone	Blood pressure
Zebeta – bisoprolol	Blood pressure
Ziac – bisoprolol	Blood pressure
Zovirax - acyclovir	Antibiotic

Medications That Have Safety Warnings

Even though medications must be tested for toxicity, safety, and therapeutic benefit before coming to market, over time some medications are found to have risks that were originally unknown. Often this is the result of certain unanticipated additional factors, such as other medications a person is currently taking, or other co-occurring biological conditions (e.g., mental illness, etc.). The following table notes currently published warnings for medications that may be contraindicated in certain situations. The federal government has also developed the Drug Watch website to provide safety information. At the time of this writing, the interim site is accessible at www.fda.gov/cder/drug/DrugSafety/DrugIndex.htm Again, of course, always check with a healthcare professional BEFORE making any changes in your medication.

Medication Safety Warnings

Substance(brand/generic)	Medication Category	Uses/ Conditions	Population at-risk	Risk Factor
Seroquel/quetiapine	Atypical antipsychotic	Psychosis/Schizophrenia	Elderly patients with dementia-related psychosis	Increased risk of death
Abilify/aripiprazole	Atypical antipsychotic	Psychosis/ Schizophrenia		Increased risk of death
Zyprexia/olanzapine	Atypical Antipsychotic	Psychosis/ Schizophrenia		Increased risk of death
Risperdal/risperidone	Atypical Antipsychotic	Psychosis/ Schizophrenia		Increased risk of death
Clozaril/clozapine	Atypical Antipsychotic	Psychosis/ Schizophrenia		Increased risk of death
Geodon/ziprasidone	Atypical Antipsychotic	Psychosis/ Schizophrenia		Increased risk of death
Symbyax/olanzapine and fluoxetine	Atypical Antipsychotic	Psychosis/ Schizophrenia		Increased risk of death
Dilantin/ Phenytoin	Anti-convulsant	Seizure disorder (thought to "boost" IQ but no evidence)	Aged	Unproven memory benefit in combination with side-

Next Step

Whew, I know that there was a lot of material presented in this chapter—much of it may be a challenge to understand as the terminology and medication names can be new to you, or a bit weird-sounding, or even daunting to understand at first, but it is all highly important and useful information. I hope you will use this section as a reference tool for deciding whether to talk to your physician about a change in your medications.

Never independently alter your dosing instructions. If you experience uncomfortable effects from any medication, contact your physician or pharmacist immediately, or if it is an emergency, CALL 911 IMMEDIENTLY. It is very important to keep all of your healthcare providers informed of all medications and supplements you are taking; any physical conditions, symptoms, or illnesses you may be experiencing, your dietary habits, and any concerns about your mental acuity. If you have concerns about any medications you are taking, you should discuss it with your prescribing healthcare professional(s). Ask the individual to explain the thinking and rational behind the treatment decision. Request being educated as to whether there may be alternative approaches, along with the pros-and-cons of each. Your pharmacist can also help you better understand your medications, their possible side effects, dosing instructions, and any other related questions as well. Doing so is your right, and any good healthcare provider should be happy to discuss these issues with you.

Chapter 7

Diet: "You Are What you Eat"

I have always liked that saying. On the one hand, it speaks to eating in a healthy fashion in order to be healthy. On the other hand, it sounds somewhat silly when considered literally (watch out for those cream puffs!). This chapter is not about going on a weight reduction diet, per se. It is about developing a diet that is sure to include healthy and nutritious ingredients and should, as a side effect, result in weight loss and a healthier younger looking body.

I have already touched upon diet, obesity, and poor nutrition in our chapter on bad habits with "The Seven Deadly Sins of Intellectual Decline." Chapter 8 will provide you with a number of exercises you can use to help with blood flow, oxygenation, lean muscle mass development, healthy joints, and so on. In Chapter 5 I gave you information on vitamin and mineral supplements that will help keep you cognitively healthy. Now I will approach nutrition and health from the most basic of aspects – your diet.

The scientific literature is filled with studies that note, for example, people who consumed 20 to 28 grams of niacin per day from the food they ate had an 80 percent reduction in Alzheimer's risk. Of course, the question remains, "What do I need to eat in order to become one of those people?" The following tables provide information on precisely that – what to eat to naturally obtain nutrients that will help promote cognitive health. Consider referring to this section from now on when you make out your grocery list.

Foods	Serving size	Vitamins/Nutrients	Helps to...
Fish	4 ounces of swordfish	13 mg of niacin	lower Alzheimer's risk and age-related cognitive decline
Cold-water fish	Salmon, mackerel, sardines (*watch out for sodium though*)	Omega-3 fatty acids	renew and maintain brain cell membranes
Poultry	4 ounces of chicken breast	15 mg of niacin	lower Alzheimer's risk and age-related cognitive decline
Low-fat dairy products	2 - 3 servings/day	Vitamin E	lower Alzheimer's risk by as much as 70%
Nuts and grains	4 - 5 servings a week	Vitamin E	lower Alzheimer's risk by ~70%

Fresh fruits and vegetables	4 - 5 servings (of each) a day	Vitamins C and E	improved antioxidant functioning to protect brain cell membranes

For some of us, it may be difficult to gain the proper amounts of nutrition solely through eating habits and dietary patterns. If this is the case for you, you may also wish to revisit Chapter 7 on nutritional supplements.

Foods To Avoid

Just as there are good things to eat to improve your mental and biological functioning, there are bad things as well that you should do your best to avoid consuming. Since this book needed to be smaller than the New York City Yellow Pages I could not list all the "bad foods" but at least I provided some top contenders for our hit list. My sincere apologies to you if any of your a favorites are listed.

Food	Why it's so bad
Raw oysters	Easily contaminated with hepatitis or other viruses
Sports Drinks	Sugar content is way too high, thus bad for your teeth and weight
Pork Rinds	Do I really have to explain this one?
Well-done steak	Charred meats are high in heterocyclic amines which are linked to cancer
Any processed lunch-meat (e.g., corned beef, pastrami, bologna)	They are loaded with saturated fats
Mayonnaise	It's been called a "dense delivery system for calories and fats"
Saturated or trans fatty acids (typically found in margarine and many baked goods)	Lowers High Density Lipoprotein (HDL), the "good" cholesterol. High consumption by those 65 and older has been associated with a doubled likelihood of developing Alzheimer's
Pop-tarts	Loaded with sugar and fat

The scientific jury is still out as to foods that actually protect your brain functioning or enhance your memory. There is robust literature on a diet that lowers your risk of other maladies that correlate with risk factors for dementia – such as diabetes, elevated homocysteine levels (an amino acid that if elevated increases the risk of heart disease as well as Alzheimer's), high blood pressure, and inflammation. Such a diet would look something like the following:

Food	At least...
Fish	3 servings a week
Vegetables (in particular, green & leafy vegetables like–spinach, & romaine lettuce, cruciferous–broccoli in particular & cauliflower)	4 - 5 servings/day (½ cup or more/day)
Fresh fruits	4 - 5 servings/day
Low-fat dairy products	2 - 3 servings/day
Nuts and beans	4 - 5 servings a week
Monounsaturated fats (as in olive oil)	2 tablespoons 4 - 5 times a week
Fiber	25 grams/day

In addition, of course, you'll need to observe the following limits:

Food	No more than...
Sodium	1500 mg/day
Sweets	5 servings/week

Next Step

Remember, "diet" is not simply limited to those focused on losing weight. Weight loss is only one issue for dieting. The point of this chapter is that adopting a consistent diet of brain-and-body-healthy foods while avoiding more seductive, less health-promoting choices will very simply help your emotional, physical, medical, and cognitive abilities and sense of well-being, and needs to become an important part of your lifestyle. If you are a vegetarian or vegan, or have food allergies or certain religious beliefs that influence your food selections, it is advisable to seek the counsel of a registered, licensed or certified healthcare professional to help you make appropriate, brain-and-body-healthy diet choices.

Chapter 8

Physical Exercises

I touched upon diet, obesity, and poor nutrition in our earlier discussion of "The Seven Deadly Sins of Intellectual Decline." I also noted the findings of a Swedish study, which found that men whose Body Mass Index (BMI) was 30 or higher, had an extraordinarily increased risk of dementia. It is worth the time to calculate your BMI and easy to do. For a website that will help you calculate your BMI go to www.nhlbisupport.com/bmi/bmicalc.htm and follow the prompts, or "simply" use the formula below:

Body Mass Index (BMI) Calculator

Your weight in pounds multiplied by 703,

then divided by your height in inches squared = BMI

or

(Number of pounds x 703) ÷ inches^2 = BMI

For example,

If you are 6'2" (74 inches) and weigh 165 pounds, then

(165 x 703) ÷ 74^2 = BMI

By working through this formula we get

115995 ÷ 5476 = a BMI of 21.2

A BMI of 25 to 29 is considered overweight. A BMI of 30 or more is obese.

Most studies of exercise and risk of Alzheimer's demonstrate a relationship such that as one goes up the other goes down or vice-versa. The problem for science is that a correlational relationship does not prove cause and effect.

Some studies suggest that regular aerobic exercise helps to maintain brain cells and stimulate new neuronal growth. It certainly helps to optimize blood pressure and develop Brain-Derived Neurotrophic Factor (BNDF) – a critically important brain protein.

Blood Pressure

Swedish researchers have found that individuals over 74 years of age who have a systolic (the top number) blood pressure that drops 15 points or more have a threefold increase in their risk of Alzheimer's Disease. Obviously, older adults in particular should have their blood pressure measured regularly.

Exercise

Whatever it is that underlies the relationship between "working out" and Alzheimer's one thing is clear: exercise and a healthier lifestyle benefit everyone. The following suggestions will vary in appropriateness for you depending on your current level of fitness, physical ability, health history, and other related factors. In either case, before beginning any physical exercise routine, first check with your physician and possibly an exercise physiologist as well for clearance and/or recommendations as to the advisability of the following for you:

Stretching

Warming and loosening your muscles at the start and end of your day can help in a number of ways. Many of us wake up with stiff muscles and joints, gently stretching can help us not only feel better, but doing so also helps you develop improved proprioception, or your brain's awareness of the positioning of your body as you move.

Frequency and duration: One or more times/day, everyday, for at least 10 to 15 minutes or more.

Walking

What more can be said for the simple and pleasurable act of walking? It is convenient, it is inexpensive (if you do not buy a $300 pair of jogging shoes), it can be done most anywhere including somewhere indoors if the weather is inclement. You can do it alone or with others, and it is very beneficial!

I suggest combining the faster, more active aerobic style of walking with a meditative, peaceful state of mind, which is facilitated by a more natural setting, such as a park. Include this as part of your regular daily walk or on alternate days.

Be sure to take a mobile phone, identification, insurance card, and cash for a taxi back in case you lose your way or twist an ankle.

Frequency and duration: Three to four times/week; work up to a mile, but if you cannot go that far when you start, be content with walking to the end of your block and back, then work up to around the block, then a few blocks, and so forth.

Yoga

Taking a yoga class suitable to your ability is a great way to learn stretching, meditative techniques, relaxation, and do so within a supportive environment of like minded others. Once you have some of the basics learned, you can do the positions at home, when traveling, anytime, anywhere. You may also want to supplement your yoga class with an instructional video from a local library or video store.

Frequency and duration: One or more times/day, everyday; 10-15 or more minutes at a time.

Strength Training

Taking a class at a local gym or fitness center on the proper techniques for training with weights can be a great way to start building lean muscle mass – no matter your age or sex. Studies have shown lifting weights appropriate to your level of fitness can help forge stronger bones, maintain or build your strength, help to burn off fat, improve overall well being, and may even help you become the governor of California..

Frequency and duration: One or more times/day, everyday; 10-15 or more minutes at a time.

Swimming/Low-impact Pool Exercises

If you have a pool or access to a pool, swimming can be a great, no-impact aerobic exercise that helps maintain cognitive abilities, build endurance and strengthen muscles.

There are also a growing number of classes offered that can teach you how to do stretches and in-water calisthenics – some with floating devices to increase resistance. All this can add to the diversity and variety of exercises in your repertoire.

Frequency and duration: One or more times/day, everyday; 10-15 or more minutes at a time.

Aerobics

Aerobics classes have been around for a long time and now offer a wide variety of activities at various skill levels – beginners, rehab, dance-styles, etc. Again, these classes offer a social opportunity as well as healthy activity. There are also a number of instructional videos that you can purchase or get at your local library for home and travel use.

Frequency: Two or more times/week.

Music and Exercise

A recent study found that listening to music while exercising actually improved mental/cognitive performance. There are many limitations to the applicability of this study across age groups and types of music, as the research only evaluated older subjects listening to Vivaldi's *The Four Seasons*. Nevertheless, adding your favorite music to your exercise routine will at least make it a more pleasurable experience, and I recommend it! I also recommend listening to soothing music, even relaxing nature sounds when not exercising.

Activities

While it is good to have some exercise-specific activities, there are a number of additional activities that you can participate in to supplement your workouts. Some research suggests that the diversity of your activities can do more to help your cognitive functioning than the intensity of your workouts. Here are some ideas for additional activities. Try them out and make habits of those that are most enjoyable to you. These include a mix of right and left-brain activities, which are also important, so get going and try to have fun!

Activities!

Bicycling	Board games
Household chores	Gardening
Mowing the lawn	Raking
Hiking	Dancing
Bowling	Golfing
Swimming	Card-playing
Reading a book	Going to a play
Going to a concert	Wandering through a museum or art gallery
Surfing the Web	Going to the movies
Playing Chess	Playing, or learning to play, an instrument

Tips and Tricks

As a clinical psychologist, I have specialized training in behavioral change. Starting and sticking with a change in behavior, like a consistent exercise plan, can be difficult without some supportive tools. One of the best ways to enjoy your accomplishments and motivate yourself for continued success is to keep a log to track your progress, whether your goal is to lose weight, build muscle mass, increase endurance, and so forth. The chart below can be used or adapted to best fit your needs. Feel free to make enough photocopies for each month and add your own targeted areas or activities.

Progress and Goals List

Month: _____	Week 1	Week 2	Week 3	Week 4	Goal
Weight					
Waist					
Thighs					
Biceps					
Distance (for walks/ run/bike)					

You can also photocopy the table below and use it to serve as a reminder and to track your progress in making exercise a regular part of your weekly routine. Show your loved ones, make the proud!

Weekly Exercise Schedule								
	Sun	Mon	Tues	Wed	Thur	Friday	Sat	Totals
Walk								
Swim								
Yoga								
Stretch								
Weights/strength								

Rest and Sleep

Appropriate sleep is also critical in maintaining health and mental focus. Deprivation studies indicate increased agitation, memory loss, and other cognitive and behavioral problems associated with the loss of sleep, especially the type of sleep during which we dream, called rapid eye movement (REM) sleep. The general rule of thumb for mental alertness is 45 minutes of sleep per 2 hours of waking time.

Needing too much sleep may indicate health problems. For example, people who sleep more than eight hours a night have a higher mortality rate than those who sleep less. Interestingly, people who sleep less than seven hours a night also have a higher mortality rate. Getting the proper amount of sleep is clearly the key in this equation.

Next Step

A final suggestion to help increase your motivation is to tell others about your new routine of exercise and activities. They may wish to join you, and that makes the process all the more enjoyable and adds a nice social aspect as well. Doing so should also more fully "commit" you to the plan as well, as your friends will then more likely ask you to go for daily walks or ask how you are doing on your program.

Keep in mind that it might be harder to get started than to keep going. Your muscles may get sore at the start. Resist the possible temptation to do too much at first. Besides cramping, doing so also increases the chance of injury, unpleasant experience, and even premature burnout! It is much better to be slow and steady at building up your miles or time. You will come to enjoy the feeling of better fitness, strength, endurance, youthfulness, well-being and BrainPower!

Chapter 9

Purpose and Quality of Life

Overview

Thinking positively and with optimism for the future, avoiding negative thoughts and people, using prayer, faith and meditation, and helping others are all factors that can contribute to improving or maintaining your cognitive abilities, physical and emotional health and, in general, your quality of life.

"Spiritual" Aspects

There is a growing body of evidence that supports the use of prayer, meditation, and other relaxation techniques to reduce and manage stress. Their impact can have measurable neurophysiological effects. One study found that attending religious activities and going to a house of worship slowed cognitive decline in individuals with Alzheimer's disease. In another study African-Americans who held a strong belief in God were less likely to be depressed than "non-believers," and depression is often a co-occurring factor in mental decline.

Meditation

Lack of focus and external pressure or status does little to help anyone's thought processes or memory. Your memory and concentration may benefit, however, if you learn and practice various meditation, relaxation, and focusing techniques. Research has shown that you can actually change your brain wave activity during meditation. There are additional benefits to increasing your sense of well-being, including reducing high blood pressure, decreasing anxiety, mitigating substance abuse, and lowering levels of cortisol (a hormone associated with the stress response). Meditation can also be in the form of prayer, which can include a chant or mantra, involving the repetition of a certain word, sound, or phrase.

Some forms of meditation are easier to learn than others. The benefits of meditation can also be derived from relaxation training, yoga, and psychotherapy as well. There are a number of similarities between these techniques, as many involve focusing particular attention on your breathing pattern. You may wish to experiment with different methods to find what works best for you. Here are some currently popular formats:

Technique	Comments
Mindfulness	This approach refers to your ability to pay attention to your experience from one moment to the next without being

distracted by other thoughts.

PMR or Progressive Muscle Relaxation	Not a meditative exercise as much as a relaxation technique, but winds up putting one in a meditative state. It involves progressively tensing and then relaxing major muscle groups.
Relaxation Response	This method uses repetition of a word or phrase or visualizing a positive mental image.

There are also classes, books, and instructional videos that can teach you how to meditate or relax. Trained behavioral psychologist also teach how meditation and relaxation techniques and their use. In the meantime, you may wish to try the following suggestion:

1) Sit, or partially recline in a comfortable position on a comfortable recliner in a quiet, dimly lit setting.

2) Once you are comfortable, focus your attention on your breathing. The best breathing technique is called abdominal or "triangular" breathing and involves inhaling deeply, paying special attention to allowing your abdomen to expand, then exhaling slowly rather than rapidly as we often do.

3) You may also want to mentally repeat a word or phrase (such as "calm" or "peace") each time you slowly exhale.

4) Allow any distracting thoughts to leave your mind as you focus on your deep, rhythmic breathing and your word or mantra.

5) Start practicing for at least 15 to 20 minutes, once or twice daily.

Work and Purpose

It is very important to maintain a sense of purpose in life. You may be retired from work, but that need not mean you have retired from life! Maybe retirement has not turned out the way you imagined it would, but that does not mean it has to stay that way. Consider volunteering or part-time work at something that attracts your interest. Help at voter registration, participate in civic meetings, visit the local library, attend a lecture–participate and contribute when possible. Especially if you were socially active in the past, continue to be a vibrant contributor to society – even if it's in ways you had not considered before. Working in retirement, even part-time, can increase the quality of your life and some studies suggest the length of it as well! Here are some resources to tap into if you are considering returning to work.

Organization	Website	Comments
The Next Chapter	www.civicventures.org	For those 55 or older looking to network and explore options
Phoenix Link	www.thephoenixlink.com	Experienced executives, resume posting opportunity
Retired Brains	www.retiredbrains.com	Part- and Full-time job listings
Senior Job Bank	www.seniorjobbank.org	Job postings for those 50 or older
YourEncore	www.yourencore.com	For experienced technical professionals such as engineers, scientists, etc.

Another approach that you may find helpful is noted in Ken Dychtwald's book, *The Power Years*. Make three lists based on the following steps:

I. Write down every job you have ever had (both volunteer and paid), and after each one list what you enjoyed most about it and when you felt the most satisfied: (You will probably need more space than I have provided)

1) _____

    a) _____

    b) _____

    c) _____

2) _____

    a) _____

    b) _____

    c) _____

3) _____

    a) _____

    b) _____

    c) _____

4) _____

    a) _____

    b) _____

    c) _____

5) _____

    a) _____

    b) _____

    c) _____

6) _____

    a) _____

    b) _____

    c) _____

7) _____

     a) _____

     b) _____

     c) _____

8) _____

     a) _____

     b) _____

     c) _____

9) _____

     a) _____

     b) _____

     c) _____

10) _____

     a) _____

     b) _____

     c) _____

II. List what you spend most of your discretionary income on:

1) _____

2) _____

3) _____

4) _____

5) _____

III. Look back over your life and list any dreams or ambitions that had to be "put on hold" due to other priorities, commitments, and obligations.

1) _____

2) _____

3) _____

4) _____

5) _____

6) _____

7) _____

8) _____

9) _____

10) _____

Next Step

Now for the fun part. Look over the three lists you just completed. The first one will help you identify satisfying aspects of your prior work that you may now wish to seek out again. The second list is likely to contain what are currently higher-level interest items for you. Things you *choose to* spend your money on. Finally, the third list is things that were important in your past and may still hold sway in your current life.

Consider all these in combination and decide what you wish to do to incorporate them into your life now and in the future. Some may be simple and short-term activities or goals, and others may be more on-going requiring years of commitment. The nice thing is you will begin to rediscover what is important to you and can take steps to enjoy those things again – and that, my friend, is the key.

Functional Activities Questionnaire (FAQ)

The Agency for Health Care Policy and Research (AHCPR)

Recommends the FAQ as particularly useful for the initial assessment of functional impairment

The FAQ is a brief, informant-based survey that evaluates performance on ten complex activities of daily living. The ten-item FAW should be administered during an interview with a knowledgeable informant – usually a family member – and is suitable for use by office staff prior to or during the physician's evaluation.

Scoring:

The patient's performance on ten items is assigned a 0 to 3 rating from independence (0=normal) to dependence (3=unable to perform independently). The total score ranges from 0 to 30, and is computed by summing the scores across the ten items.

Points	Patient's Performance in Each Activity
3	Completely unable to perform
2	Requires Assistance
1	Has difficulty but accomplishes task, or
	Has never done task; however, informant feels patient could accomplish it, but with difficulty
0	Normal performance, or
	Has never done task, but informant feels patient could do so now

Interpretation:

A score of 9 or more, showing dependency in three or more activities, is an indication of functional impairment sufficient to consider a more complete diagnostic evaluation. The degree of change over time and the speed of functional change are important considerations for the clinician in the evaluation of function as it relates to a dementia diagnosis.

Next Steps:

Performance on this questionnaire does not establish criteria for dementia, but can be useful in determining whether further cognitive evaluations are necessary, and a complete diagnostic evaluation for dementia should be considered. This evaluation should include a standardized cognitive assessment scale such as the Mini-Mental State Examination (MMSE).

Functional Activities

Questionnaire (FAQ)*

Observer's name: _____

Patient's name: _____

Date: _____

Instructions:

Place a check mark under the column that best describes the patient's ability to perform the tasks listed below:

	(3 points)	(2 points)	(1 point)	(0 points)
1. Writing checks, paying bills, balancing a checkbook	_____	_____	_____	_____
2. Assembling tax records, business affairs, or papers	_____	_____	_____	_____
3. Shopping alone for clothes, house-hold necessities, or groceries	_____	_____	_____	_____
4. Playing a game of skill, working on a hobby	_____	_____	_____	_____
5. Heating water, making a cup of coffee, turning off the stove	_____	_____	_____	_____
6. Preparing a balanced meal keeping track of current				

events	_____	_____	_____	_____
7. Paying attention to, understanding, discussing a TV show, book, or magazine	_____	_____	_____	_____
8. Remembering appointments, family occasions, holidays, medications	_____	_____	_____	_____
9. Traveling out of the neighborhood, driving, arranging to take buses	_____	_____	_____	_____
Points per column	_____	_____	_____	_____

Total Points _____

*Adapted from J. Pfeffer, RI, Kurosaki IT, Harrah CH Jr., et. Al. *Measurement of Functional Activities of Older Adults in the Community.* J Gerontol. 1982; 37: 323-329.

Appendix B

Extended Personal Inventory

Additional information to share with your doctors

Current Symptoms Check List

How is your appetite?

_____

Do you eat 3 or more meals per day? _____

Do you eat healthy, balanced meals? _____

Do you keep yourself hydrated? _____

How are you sleeping? _____

Do you wake up frequently? _____

Do you fall asleep easily? _____

Do you have bowel or bladder issues? _____

      If yes, please describe: _____

Have you ever suffered a head trauma, loss of consciousness, or seizures? If yes, please describe in more detail.

_____

_____

What were your various occupations?

_____

What illnesses or accidents have you had (list all and your age when they occurred)?

_____

_____

_____

What languages did you speak or understand as a child? _____

Can you still understand and speak them? _____

What kinds of movies, books and music appealed to you when you were young, growing up, and now?

_____
_____

Were you ever married and/or in a long relationship?

_____

Did you have or raise children?_____

Are you in touch with your children, or relatives or friends?_____

Were you social at some periods in your life, and not in others?

_____

Were you ever separated or divorced? _____

Did you have to deal with sick or dying parents, spouses or relatives?

_____

Were you ever treated or hospitalized for emotional reasons and, if so, what kinds of treatment did you have? _____

Were you ever in trouble with the law or have to go to court?

_____

Were you ever a ward of the state, raised by people other than your folks, raised in a state facility.*_____

Emotional Signs and Symptoms

Do you feel depressed? _____

Do you feel anxious? _____

Do you feel angry (often?)_____

Do you experience mood swings?_____

Do you think of suicide? _____

Do you think of killing someone else? _____

Do you feel people or things are against you or after you? _____

Do you feel that you have special powers? _____

Do you feel that you are blessed, cursed, lucky, or unlucky? _____

Do you feel that the world is against you, has abandoned you or that you have been singled out for special punishment or a special positive destiny?_____

Do you feel out of touch with the world around you? _____

Are you lonely, alone, or do you feel helpless, hopeless and worthless?
_____

Do you feel that the radio, TV or computer is rigged, bugged, or is influencing you?
_____

Do shapes and sound seem to change at times?_____

Do you use alcohol? _____

How frequently do you use alcohol? _____

How much alcohol do you consume? _____

Do you use illicit substances? _____

Have you ever been arrested for a DUI? _____ When? _____

Are you on any psychotropic medication now? _____

Have you ever been on such medication?_____

Social History

Were you born in the United States? Yes ___ No ___ If not, where were you born and how old were you when you came to America?
_____
_____

Schooling (e.g. grammar school, high school, jr. college, college, trade school, military training – service, rank, MO, dates of service, did you see combat, discharge type, ever wounded, ever demoted, ever punished, equivalent for foreign service, on the job training or equivalent for Europe, Asian or North or South America).
_____
_____

Learning Styl.

Did you have difficulty in school/receive special educational services? If yes please describe in detail.

_____
_____
_____

Interpersonal History

Were you ever diagnosed with ADD/ADHD or other type of learning disability?
Yes ___ No ___ If yes please describe:_____

Did you ever have conflicts with authority figures?_____

Did you ever have conflicts with spouses or in dating relationships?

_____
_____

Do you prefer to be alone?_____

Do you feel you need assistance/help?_____

What areas do you need assistance/help with?_____

Have there been any changes in your ability to manage daily activities? If yes, please describe in detail.

_____
_____
_____

Parents' health/mental health history. Describe in detail.

_____
_____
_____
_____
_____

Glossary

Acetylcholine – a neurotransmitter crucial to memory and learning

Adequate intake (AI) – an estimate for the nutritional needs of healthy people used when there are not enough data to support an RDA.

ADmark Assays – two clinical tests for Alzheimer's disease. One measure beta-amyloaid and tau protein in the spinal fluid; the other tests for the apolipoprotein E e4 genotype.

Age-associated memory impairment – normal forgetfulness that increases with age.

Alzheimer's disease – a progressive disorder of the brain that is characterized by deterioration of mental faculties resulting from the loss of nerve cells and the connections between them. Also called Alzheimer disease.

Amnestic syndrome – severe memory loss despite maintenance of normal intelligence.

Amyloid plaques – dense deposits of beta-amyloid pieces of damaged nerve cells, and other proteins. Found in the brains of virtually all people with Alzheimer's disease.

Amyloid precursor protein – a protein that is split in two by enzymes to produce beta-amyloid.

Antioxidant – a substance that helps protect the body against destructive free radicals and other unstable molecules by giving up electrons. Antioxidant micronutrients include beta carotene and other carotenoids, vitamin C, and vitamin E.

Aphasia – A partial or complete inability to use or understand language.

Apolipoprotein E (APOE) – a gene on chromosome 19. The e4 version of this gene is associated with an increased risk of Alzheimer's disease.

Beta-amyloid – a sticky, starch-like protein that is the main component of amyloid plaques.

Beta-carotene – a precursor that is converted by the body into vitamin A. Beta carotene acts as an anti-oxidant. It's found in many green vegetables and dark yellow or deep orange fruits and vegetables.

Bioavailability – how quickly and how completely a nutrient can be absorbed and used by the body.

Bone mineral density – the amount of mineralized bone tissue in a given area, usually calculated in grams per square centimeter.

Carotenoids – plant and animal pigments that color many fruits and vegetables, including carrots and cantaloupe. Some carotenoids can be converted to vitamin A.

Cerebellum – a fist-sized structure, located at the base of the brain beneath the cerebral cortex, that coordinates movement and balance.

Cerebral cortex – the convoluted outer layer of gray matter that constitutes the "thinking" portion of the brain.

Choline – a substance used by the body to produce acetylcholine. Present in food.

Cholinesterase inhibitors – medications that slow the breakdown of acetylcholine. Used in the treatment of Alzheimer's disease.

Colchicine – an anti-inflammatory drug commonly used to treat gout. Currently being tested as a treatment for Alzheimer's disease.

Complete blood cell count – measures cellular elements of blood; red blood cells, white blood cells, and platelets. Helps rule out anemia, infections, and vitamin B12 deficiency as causes of dementia or factors that can exacerbate dementia.

Computed tomography (CT) – an imaging technique that uses x-rays to create a two-dimensional image of the brain or other parts of the body.

Creutzfeldt-Jakob disease (CJD) – a rare, fatal brain disorder that causes a rapid, progressive dementia. Sometimes mistaken for Alzheimer's disease.

Cushing's disease – A disorder resulting from the overproduction of hormones by the adrenal gland.

Daily value (DV) – A measurement, found on the "Nutrition Facts" labels of packaged food, that reports the amounts of specific micronutrients and other key dietary components per serving, stated as a percentage of daily requirements. DV's do not take life stages into account, but instead reflect the highest amount of a nutrient an individual might need.

Dementia – a significant intellectual decline or impairment that persists over time in several areas of thinking.

Dementia with Lewy bodies – A type of dementia characterized by episodes of confusion, falls, and repetitive hallucinations, as well as signs of parkinsonism early in the disease.

Dietary reference intakes (DRI's) – a comprehensive set of new standards for essential vitamins and minerals based on evidence from scores of observational and clinical studies.

Dietary supplements - vitamins, minerals, herbs, amino acids, enzymes, organ tissues, and a few other substances promoted as a way to bolster diet. Unlike drugs, they are not regulated by the FDA.

Estimated average requirement (EAR) - the daily amount of a given nutrient estimated to meet the nutritional need of half the healthy people in a specific life stage group. EAR's are used to help scientific panels determine RDA's and AI's.

Fat-soluble vitamins - a group of organic substances essential for human life; includes vitamins A, D, E, and K. In the body, fat-soluble vitamins are stored in the fat tissues and liver.

Flavonoid - an antioxidant substance found in tea, berries, tomatoes, and onions, among other sources.

Free radicals - unstable molecules that can alter DNA, oxidize LDL cholesterol, and damage cells and tissues throughout the body by stealing electrons. Free radicals are implicated in aging, cataracts, cancer, and heart disease, among other ills.

Frontotemporal dementia - a spectrum of disorders associated with impaired initiation of plans and goal setting, personality changes, language difficulties, and unawareness of any loss of mental function.

Gray matter - the area of the brain, gray in appearance, that contains cell bodies (as opposed to white matter, which contains the nerve fibers that extend from the cell bodies).

Hemochromatosis - an excess of iron that may damage body tissues and raise risks for infection, heart disease, liver cancer, and arthritis. Causes include a genetic glitch, large doses of iron supplements, multiple blood transfusions, alcoholism, and some rare metabolic disorders.

Hippocampus - a small, S-shaped structure in the brain that appears to play a major role in the process of forging memories.

Huntington's Disease - a rare, hereditary disorder of the central nervous system characterized by uncontrollable movements and dementia.

Incontinence - an inability to control urination or defecation.

Lecithin - a substance used by the body to produce acetylcholine. Occurs naturally in food.

Lewy bodies - abnormal structures that are found in cells throughout the brain in people with dementia with Lewy bodies.

Life stage – categories used in the DRI's that group people by age, sex, and other characteristics likely to affect nutrient needs.

Long-term memory – holds information that was learned as recently as a few minutes ago and as long ago as early childhood.

Magnetic resonance imagine (MRI) – an imaging technique that uses a powerful magnet, rather than x-rays, to create a two-dimensional image of various areas of the body, including the brain.

Major minerals – a group of inorganic substances essential for human life; includes calcium, phosphorus, potassium, sulphur, sodium, chloride, and magnesium. Major minerals can appear in the body in amounts of up to a pound or slightly more.

Micronutrients – nutrients such as vitamins and minerals that the body requires in fairly small quantities.

Mild cognitive impairment (MCI) –forgetfulness that is worse than normal for one's age but is not associated with certain cognitive problems common in dementia, such as disorientation or confusion. Severity falls between age-associated memory impairment and early dementia.

Mini-Mental State Examination – a test of mental status used to screen for basic cognitive impairment.

Neurofibrillary tangles – found in the brains of virtually all people with Alzheimer's disease. Composed mainly of the protein tau. Appear as twist3ed, hair-like threads and remain after the collapse of the microtubules in the nerve cell.

Neuron – nerve cell.

Neurotransmitter – a specialized chemical that relays messages between nerve cells.

Nonsteroidal anti-inflammatory drugs (NSAIDs) – a class of drugs, commonly used to treat arthritis, which may be effective in the treatment and prevention of Alzheimer's disease.

Normal-pressure hydrocephalus – a condition characterized by excess fluid in the brain that can result in dementia.

Oxalates – substances in fibre, beets, rhubarb, and spinach that bind with calcium so the body cannot absorb it.

Parkinson's disease – a progressive neurological disease characterized by tremors, stooped posture, slow movement, poor balance, and shuffling gait.

Phytates – substances in whole grains, legumes, and seeds that bind with certain micronutrients such as iron, calcium, magnesium, copper, and zinc, so that they pass through the intestines instead of being absorbed and used by the body.

Phytochemicals – compounds in plants that affect their taste, color, scent, and other properties. Lycopene, found in tomatoes, is one phytochemical thought to have beneficial effects for humans.

Pick's disease – a type of frontotemporal dementia characterized by impaired initiation of plans and goal setting, personality changes, unawareness of any loss of mental function, and language difficulties.

Piracetam – a steroid drug with powerful anti-inflammatory effects. Currently being tested as a treatment for Alzheimer's disease.

Precursor – a substance that the body can convert into the active form of a vitamin. One example is beta carotene, which the body can convert into vitamin A as needed.

Prions – unusual infectious agents that cause Creutzfeldt-Jakob disease.

Recommended dietary allowance (RDA) – the average daily amount of a micronutrient that will meet the nutritional needs of almost all (97%-98%) healthy people at specific stages of their lives.

Selegiline – a medication used to treat Parkinson's disease that is currently being tested as a therapy for Alzheimer's disease. It has antioxidant effects similar to vitamin E but is associated with more side effects.

Short-term memory – also known as working memory. Sometimes equated with consciousness.

Subdural hematoma – a collection of blood between the skull and the brain that can lead to memory problems and loss of consciousness.

Tolerable upper intake level (UL) – the highest amount of a nutrient deemed likely to have no harmful health effects for almost all healthy people when taken consistently. When people take more than the UL, the risk for ill effects rises along with the dose.

Trace minerals – a group of inorganic substances essential for life, includes iron, zinc, copper, manganese, iodine, selenium, fluoride, chromium, and molybdenum. Trace minerals appear in the body in exceedingly tiny amounts.

Vascular dementia – a disorder, often resulting from a series of tiny strokes in the brain, that can lead to dementia.

Vasopressin – a hormone produced by the hypothalamus and used as an alternative treatment to enhance memory.

Water-soluble vitamins – a group of organic substances, present in the watery portions of foods, essential to sustaining life; includes thiamine (vitamin B1), riboflavin (vitamin B2), niacin (vitamin B), biotin, pantothenic acid, vitamin B6, folic acid, vitamin B12, and vitamin C.

References and Resources

Articles

Alzheimer's seen as peril to even more, Kotulak, R. (8 March 2005). Chicago Tribune, pp 1, 24.

Benefits and risks of vitamins and minerals. Stampfer, M. J. (2005). Harvard Health Publications: Boston, MA.

Best bets in preventing Alzheimer's, April, 2005, University of California, Berkeley Wellness Letter, 21 (7), pp. 1 - 2.

Brain healthy strategies, June, 2005, The Johns Hopkins Medical Letter, Health After 50. pp. 1 - 2.

Can PET Scan help diagnose Alzheimer's disease? 2005, The Johns Hopkins Medical Letter, Health After 50, pp. 1 - 2.

Cacioppo JT, et al. (2002). Loneliness and health: Potential mechanisms. <u>Psychosomatic Medicine</u>, 64: 407-417.

Colcombe SJ, et al. (2003). Aerobic fitness reduces brain tissue loss in aging humans. <u>Journals of Gerontology Series A: Biological Sciences and Medical Sciences</u>, 58: M176-M180.

Dementia: Delaying its onset, slowing its progression, March, 2005, Mayo Clinic Health Letter, p. 7.

Dementia: Risks of using versus not using atypical antipsychotics, 4 (8), Current in Psychiatry, pp. 15, 17, 22 - 24, 27- 28.

Duke J, et al. (2002). Giving up and replacing activities in response to illness. <u>Journal of Gerontology</u>, 57B(4): P367-P376.

Improving Memory, A. Nelson and W. S. Albert, 2004, Harvard Health Publications: Boston, MA.

Kohut M, et al. (2002). Exercise and psychosocial factors modulate immunity to influenza vaccine in elderly individuals. <u>Journal of Gerontology</u>, 57A(9): M557-M562.

Meditation: Tuning the mind to help heal the body, 2003, Mayo Clinic Letter, 23 (3), pp. 4 - 5.

Mind over misery, 2005, The Futurist, July/August, 14 - 15.

Morrow-Howell N, et al. (2003). Effects of volunteering on the well-being of older adults. Journal of Gerontology, 58B(3): S137–S145.

Nutrition and brain power. McKhann, G. and Albert, M. (2005). The Johns Hopkins Medical Institutions Special Reports, The Memory Bulletin, pp. 1 - 6.

Ott A, et al. (2004). Effect of smoking on global cognitive function in nondemented elderly. Neurology, 62: 920–924.

Participation in cognitively stimulating activities and risk of incident Alzheimer disease, Wilson, R. A. et al (2002). JAMA, February 13, 2002, 287 (6) pp. 742 - 748.

Quick head check, Men's Health, July/August, 2005, p. 62,

Segerstrom SC, et al. (1998). Optimism is associated with mood, coping, and immune change in response to stress. Journal of Personality and Social Psychology, 74(6): 1646–1655.

Seshadri, S. et al (14 February 2002). Plasma homocysteine as a risk factor for dementia and Alzheimer's disease. NEJM, 346 (7), pp. 476 - 483.

Sleeping and Aging, September, 2005, Mayo Clinic Health Letter, p. 6.

Staying well, 2005, Consumer Reports on Health, p. 1, 4 - 5.

Tamar Haspel, The super diet, Men's Health, July/August, 2005, pp. 114, 117.

U.S. Department of Health and Human Services (1996). Physical Activity and Health: A Report of the Surgeon General Executive Summary. Available online: http://www.fitness.gov/execsum.htm.

Variety boosts brain-shielding benefits of exercise, August, 2005, Consumer Reports on Health, p. 10.

Wellness Facts, University of California, Berkeley Wellness Letter, 21 (12), September 2005, p. 1.

Yaffe K, et al. (2001). A prospective study of physical activity and cognitive decline in elderly women. Archives of Internal Medicine, 161: 1703–1708.

Brain Injury Workbook, T. Powell and K. Malia, 2004, Speechmark: Oxon, UK.

Braverman, E.R. *The Edge Effect.* 2004, Sterling Publishing: NY.

Fortgang, L.B., *Living Your Best Life.* 2001. Penguin Putnam, Inc. New York.

Greenstein, S. Davidson, H.E. (Eds). *A Pocket Guide to Dementia and Associated Behavioral*

Symptoms: Diagnosis, Assessment, and Management, Second Edition, 2003. Developed by Insight Therapeutics, LLC, Supported through an unrestricted educational grant from Abbott Labs. Access Medical Group, Department of Continuing Medical Education:, Arlington Heights, IL.

Handbook of Dementia, P. A. Lichtenberg, D. L. Murman, and A. N. Mellow, 2003 , John Wiley and Sons: Hoboken, NJ.

Improving Your Memory, J. Fogler and L. Stern, 2005, Johns Hopkins University Press: Baltimore MD.

Mason, D.J., and M. L. Kohn. 2001. *The Memory Workbook.* Oakland, Calif.: New Harbinger Publications.

Mason, D.J. and S.X. Smith. 2005. *Memory Doctor.* Oakland, Calif.: New Harbinger Publications.

Mason, D.J., Smith, S.X. *Memory Doctor,* 2005, New Harbinger Publications: Oakland CA.

Mason, D.J., Kohn, M.L. Memory Workbook, D. J. Mason and M. L. Kohn, 2001, New Harbinger Publications: Oakland CA.

Mayo Clinic – Staying Mentally Sharp, Mayo Clinic Health Information, 2004, Mayo Foundation: Rochester, MN.

PDR Guide to Drug Interactions, Side Effects, and Indications. 2006. Thompson Healthcare, Florence, KY.

PDR for Nonprescription Drugs, Dietary Supplements, and Herbs. 2006. Thompson Healthcare, Florence, KY.

PDR for Herbal Medicines, Third Edition. 2004. Thompson Healthcare, Florence, KY.

PDR Drug Guide for Mental Health Professionals, Second Edition. 2004, Thompson Healthcare, Florence, KY.

Physician's Desk Reference. 2000-2006. Thomason PDR: Montvale, New Jersey.

Physician's Guide to Alternative Medicine, volume VII.

Picture Perfect Prescription, H. Shapiro, 2005, Chamberlain Brothers: NY.

Pizzorno, I.U., Pizzorno, J.E. II and Murray, M.T. *Natural Medicine Instructions for Patients.* 2002

Practical Dementia Care , Rabins, P. V. et al (1999). Oxford University Press.

Preston, J.D., J.H. O'Neil, and M.E. Talaga. 1999. *Handbook of Clinical Psychopharmacology for Therapists.* 2nd edition. Oakland, Calif.: New Harbinger Publications.

R. Peterson (ed.), Mayo Clinic on Alzheimer's Disease. 2002, Mayo Foundation: Rochester, MN.

Real Vitamin and Mineral Book, S. Lieberman and N. Bruning, 1993, Avery: NY.

Retraining Cognition, R Parente and D. Herrmann, 2003, Pro-Ed: Austin, TX.

Textbook of Natural Medicine. Third Edition, 2006. St. Louis, MO. Churchill Livingstone Elsevine Ltd.

The 36-Hour Day, N. L. Mace and P. V. Rabins, 1999, Warner Books: NY.

Treating Memory Impairments, V. S. Dohrmann, 1994, Pro-Ed: Austin, TX.

Websites

Nutrition and Supplements

Computer Access to Research on Dietary Supplements (CARDS)
http://dietary-supplements.info.nih.gov/Research/CARDS_Database.aspx

Tufts University Nutrition Information website
www.navigator.tufts.edu

Organizations

Alcoholics Anonymous
www.alcoholics-anonymous.org

Alzheimer's Association
800-272-3900
www.alz.org

Alzheimer's Disease Education and Referral Center
800-438-4380
www.alzheimers.org

Alzheimer's Disease Research/American Health Assistance Foundation
800-437-2423
www.ahaf.org

American Geriatric Society Foundation for Health and Aging
800-563-4916
www.healthinaging.org

American Psychiatric Association
703-907-7300
www.psych.org

American Psychological Association
800-374-2721
www.apa.org

American Stroke Association
800-553-6321
www.strokeassociation.org

Association for the Care of Children's Health (ACCH)
-raising a child or adolescent with a disability or chronic illness

609-224-1742
www.acch.org

Attention Deficit Hyperactivity Disorder Assocation
482-945-2101
www.add.org

Autism Network International
www.ani.autistics.org

Autism Society of America
301-657-0881
www.autism-society.org

Brain Injury Association of America
800-444-6443
www.biansa.org

Children and Adults with Attention Deficit and Hyperactivity Disorder (CHADD)
800-233-4050
www.chadd.org

Food and Drug Administration
888-463-6332
www.cfsan.fda.gov

International Dyslexia Association
410-296-0232
www.interdys.org

Learning Disabilities Association of America
412-341-1515
www.ldaamerica.org
National Academy of Sciences
202-334-2000
www.nas.edu/nrc

National Aphasia Association
800-922-4622
www.aphasia.org

National Center for Complementary and Alternative Medicine
888-644-6226
www.nccam.nih.gov

National Dietetic Association
312-899-0040
www.eatright.org

National Eldercare Locator
800-677-1116
www.eldercare.gov

National Institute on Aging Information Center
800-222-2225
www.nia.nih.gov

National Institute of Mental Health
866-615-6464
www.nimh.nih.gov

National Institute of Neurological Disorders and Stroke
800-352-9424
www.ninds.nih.gov

National Mental Health Association
800-969-6642
www.nmha.org

Older Women's League (OWL)
800-825-3695
www.owl-national.org

Smoke Enders
http://www.smokenders.com

Quit smoking guide
www.quit-smoking-guide.com/quit-smoking-product-reviews.htm

Other Materials

Healthy Aging brochure, free, 877.692.4464

Sabiston, D.S., ed. 1997. Alzheimer's Disease. *Duke Medical Update* 4(1)

The Johns Hopkins White Papers–Memory, P. V. Rabins and S. Margolis, 2004, Johns Hopkins School of Medicine: Baltimore, MD.

The Memory Bulletin, Fall, 2004, Johns Hopkins School of Medicine: Baltimore, MD.

The Memory Bulletin, Winter 2004/2005, Johns Hopkins School of Medicine: Baltimore, MD.

The Memory Bulletin, Spring 2005, Johns Hopkins School of Medicine: Baltimore.

Author's Biography

Dr. Chris Stout is a licensed clinical psychologist and has a diverse background in various domains. He is the Founding Director of the Center for Global Initiatives (CenterForGlobalInitiatives.org) which was ranked as a **Top Healthcare Nonprofit** by GreatNonprofits.org (2011). His entrepreneurial experience is demonstrated in multiple start-ups that include the areas of financial management, healthcare centers, engineering, two dot-coms, real estate, and executive coaching (with a top-tier client list that includes Oracle). He also is a Clinical Full Professor in the College of Medicine, Department of Psychiatry; an Advisory Board Member to the College of Medicine's Center for Global Health; a Fellow in the School of Public Health Leadership Institute, and is a Core Faculty at the International Center on Responses to Catastrophes at the University of Illinois, Chicago. He also holds an academic appointment in the Northwestern University Feinberg Medical School, Department of Psychiatry and Behavioral Sciences' Mental Health Services and Policy Program, and was a Visiting Professor in the Department of Health Systems Management at Rush University. He served as a Non-Governmental Organization Special Representative to the United Nations. He was appointed by the Secretary of the US Department of Commerce to the Board of Examiners for the Baldrige National Quality Award. He is on the Advisory Board of the American Board of Independent Medical Examiners, and numerous other organizations. He holds the distinction of being one of only 100 world-wide leaders appointed to the World Economic Forum's Global Leaders of Tomorrow 2000 – joining the ranks of Tony Blair, Jody Foster, Bill Gates, R. J. Rowling, and Lance Armstrong, and he was an Invited Faculty at the Annual Meeting in Davos. He was invited by the Club de Madrid and Safe-Democracy to serve on the Madrid-11 Countering Terrorism Task Force. He is the founder of GordianKnot, LLC, an executive leadership consultancy and he currently runs Research and Development for a national sports and rehabilitation medicine organization with $300M in annual revenues.

Dr. Stout is a Fellow in three Divisions of the American Psychological Association, past-President of the Illinois Psychological Association, and is a Distinguished Practitioner in the National Academies of Practice. He was appointed as a Special (Citizen) Ambassador and Delegation Leader to South Africa and Eastern Europe by the Eisenhower Foundation. He serves as Acquisitions Editor for the *Journal of Disability Medicine*, and is the Series Editor of *Contemporary Psychology* (Praeger) and *"Getting Started"* (Wiley & Sons). He produced the critically acclaimed four volume set *The Psychology of Terrorism* and more recently, the highly praised and award–winning three volume set, *The New Humanitarians*, and is an Amazon.com Best Selling Author (reaching a #11 ranking). Additionally, he has published or presented over 300 papers and 30 books/manuals on various topics in psychology, including the popular *Evidence-Based Practice* (Wiley & Sons, 2005, with R. Hayes). His works have been translated into 8 languages. He has lectured across the nation and internationally in over 20 countries, and visited 6 continents and over 80 countries. He was noted as being *"one of the most frequently cited psychologists in the scientific literature"* in a study by Hartwick College. He is the 2004 winner of the American Psychological Association's International Humanitarian Award, the 2006 recipient of the Illinois

Psychological Association's Humanitarian Award, the 2008 recipient of the Psychologists for Social Responsibility's Humanitarian Award, and the 2009 winner of APA's Division on International Psychology's Outstanding Psychologist Award. He is an inaugural Inductee into his high school's, Purdue University's, and the American Motorcyclist Association's Hall of Fame.

He has served as Chief of Psychology, Director of Research, and Senior VP of an integrated behavioral healthcare system during a 15 year tenure. He served as Illinois' first Chief of Psychological Services for the Department of Human Services/Division of Mental Health–having made him the highest ranking psychologist in the State of Illinois and a committed reformer of psychology within the governmental setting. He also served as Chief Clinical Information Officer for the State's Division of Mental Health in 2004–a Cabinet-level position. He is the first psychologist to have an invited appointment to the Lake County Board of Health. The breadth of his work ranges from having served as a judge for Dean Kamen's FIRST Robotics competitions, to serving on the Young Leaders Forum of the Chicago Community Trust. His humanitarian activities include going on international missions with the Flying Doctors of America to Vietnam, Rwanda, Peru, and the Amazon; War Child in Russia; having worked with the Kovler Center (for Refugee Survivors of Torture), Amnesty International, RWJ Foundation, the Elizabeth Morse Charitable Trust, and Psychologists for Social Responsibility. He founded a kindergarten for AIDS orphaned children in Tanzania and continues as a consultant. He also was a delegate at the State of the World Forum in Belfast. He is a signatory to the UN's 50th Anniversary of the Universal Declaration of Human Rights. He is the inventor of the *"52 Ways to Change the World"* card deck. He is listed in *Fast Co.'s* Global Fast 50 nominees and in TED Conferences Founder Richard Saul Wurman's *"Who's Really Who, 1000: The Most Creative Individuals in America."* He currently serves on the Illinois Disaster Mental Health Coalition, the Medical Reserve Corp, and he is a member of the APA Disaster Response Network. He has won awards for public service announcements he's written and produced as well as for his photography—one was displayed in the Smithsonian.

Dr. Stout was educated at Purdue, The University of Chicago's Graduate School of Business, and Forest Institute, gaining over twenty-four awards and four scholarships; including, the Purdue Distinguished Academic Performance Award, the Purdue Alumni Association Distinguished Service Award, and Valedictorian of his doctoral class. He obtained post-doctoral experience at Harvard Medical School as a Fellow in neuro-developmental behavioral pediatrics. He received his second doctorate in clinical psychology as an honorific from Argosy University in recognition for his contributions to the fields of medicine and healthcare. He was awarded "Distinguished Alumni of the Year from Purdue University" in 1991, Federal Advocacy awards from AAP (1997) and APA (1998), APA's Heiser Award (1999), and IPA's Distinguished Psychologist of the Year (1999) in addition to over 30 other post-doctoral awards.

He has been interviewed on many radio, cable, local, and national television programs (e.g., CNBC, CNN, WGN, NBC, PBS, NPR, Medical Rounds, Chicago Tonight,

CL-TV, Oprah, Eye On Harvard, Christina, Bertise Berry, et al), and by numerous publications (*Time, Chicago Tribune, The Wall Street Journal, New York Times, USA Today, Women's Day, Modern Healthcare, Associated Press, Child Magazine, Chicago Sun-Times, Windy City Sports, NorthShore Magazine, Monitor on Psychology*, ...). He coined the term *"Emmortality"* and numerous registered service-marks. He was an American Delegate and presenter at the 1st International Conference on Unconventional Computing. A unique and distinct honor was his being named one of ten Volunteer's of the Year by *Pioneer Press* in 1999, for his global efforts, and both the Senate and House similarly recognized his work by proclamation of "Dr. Chris E. Stout Week."

His current interests are in the multidisciplinary aspects of global psychology and healthcare, complex systems, evidence-based practice, and battling mediocrity. He's an avid endurance- and adventure-sportsman as an ultra-marathon runner, certified diver (Blue Hole, Great Barrier Reef, narco- and shark-dives), and an devoted (albeit amateur) alpinist, having thus far summited 3 of the world's 7 Summits as well as Mt. Whitney (tallest in 49 states), Mt. Rainier, Yosemite's Half-Dome, and he founded SummitsForOthers.org, much of which is documented in his forthcoming book **"A Life In Full:** *The* **List of A Lifetime."** He also shows concours-winning vintage BMW motorcycles and Porsches as well as builds custom café racers, but his greatest joy comes from being with his best friend and wife, Dr. Karen Beckstrand and their two children, Grayson and Annika.

Contact him at: TheListOfALifetime@gmail.com   847.550.0092   ALifeInFull.org

APA International Humanitarian Award Winner

Citation: "For his tireless pioneering of cross-disciplinary projects world-wide, in healthcare, medical education and sciences, human rights, poverty, conflict, policy, sustainable development, diplomacy, and terrorism, all of which result in a tapestry with psychology serving as the integrating thread, we honor Dr. Chris Edward Stout. He is a rare individual who takes risks, stimulates new ideas, and enlarges possibilities in areas of great need but few resources. He is able to masterfully navigate between the domains of policy development while also rolling-up his sleeves to provide in-the-trenches care. His drive and vigor are disguised by his quick humor and ever-present kindness. He is provocative in his ideas and evocative in spirit. His creative solutions and inclusiveness crosses conceptual boundaries as well physical borders. No one is more deserving of this highest recognition than our esteemed colleague, Dr. Chris Edward Stout, whose work and impact spans the globe."

Psychology's Rock Star

Monitor on Psychology, December 2007, Vol 38, No. 11, page 41

It's the rare psychologist who gets to trade intellectual bon mots with international luminaries such as Bono, Al Gore, Tony Blair, *both* Clintons and Steve Jobs. But, after

Chris E. Stout, PsyD, was named one of the World Economic Forum's 100 Global Leaders for Tomorrow in 2000—a group of world leaders under age 40 who have demonstrated socially responsible leadership—he was invited to the World Economic Forum in Davos, Switzerland, for three years running.

"You never really know why you get invited," jokes Stout. "My impression was that it was a mistake."

But there's no mistaking Stout's passion for integrating psychology with public health around the world. Since the early '90s, Stout has been bringing health and psychological assistance to children and families in countries such as Vietnam, Rwanda and Peru. Building on his former work as a child psychologist, his involvement in global health projects, the time he spent at the United Nations as part of APA's nongovernmental organization and the connections he made in Davos, Stout founded the Center for Global Initiatives in 2004 to train health-care professionals and students to create sustainable programs.

"We develop projects that can be handed off to locals," says Stout. The center's projects have included establishing a kindergarten in Tanzania for children orphaned by AIDS and providing health care to families living in Bolivian prisons.

Most recently, Stout brought a group of nurses, physicians and other health professionals to the center to design a project to train groups of Cambodian villagers in basic emergency medicine and first aid that can be used to stabilize injured people until they can get to a hospital.

Stout has further plans for the Bolivian prisons, where inmates' children live and go to school when there's no one else on the outside to care for them. The teachers there have no resources, so Stout is assembling child-friendly psychological and resiliency materials, children's books and parenting information. He plans to use center funds to send interested psychology grad students to the prisons to train the teachers to incorporate the materials.

Not as glamorous as Davos, but exactly where Stout wants to be.